ASTHMA

The Complete Guide to Self-Management of Asthma and Allergies for Patients and Their Families

Allan M. Weinstein, M.D.

FAWCETT CREST • NEW YORK

Although this book is designed to assist you to better understand and deal with asthma, it is not intended to be a substitute for the ongoing care of your own personal physician. The author and publisher disclaim any responsibility for any adverse effects resulting from the information programs or management suggestions presented in this book, and urge you to consult your personal physician before implementing any of the information contained herein.

A Fawcett Crest Book
Published by Ballantine Books
Copyright © 1987 by Allan M. Weinstein, M.D.

Drawings and tables created by Artisan Graphics, Alexandria, Virginia

Library of Congress Catalog Card Number: 86-10574

ISBN 0-449-21562-8

This edition published by arrangement with McGraw-Hill Book Company, a division of McGraw-Hill, Inc.

Manufactured in the United States of America

First Ballantine Books Edition: May 1988
Tenth Printing: January 1992

For Linda, David, and Jessica

◇ **Acknowledgments** ◇

For their detailed review of the manuscript, I would like to acknowledge and thank my mentors: my brother Dr. Robert Weinstein, who is an allergist in private practice in Southfield, Michigan, and Dr. Michael Kaliner, Head of the Allergy Section of the National Institutes of Health in Bethesda, Maryland.

Special thanks are due to my dear friend Joshua Javits for his encouragement and help in initiating this project.

I acknowledge my indebtedness to my many professors and colleagues at the National Jewish Center for Immunology and Respiratory Medicine in Denver, Colorado, and at the National Institutes of Health.

I also wish to thank my office staff for their understanding, and my patients for the many things they have taught me.

My thanks are due to the following people who have helped me in so many different ways: Barbara and Albert LaPlume, Lucy Seifert, Melissa Talley, Patti Wunderley, Suzanne Crichton, Maureen Gillen, Coretta Pattison, Beatriz Cadme, Arie Duvall, and Vinod Ajmani and his staff at Artisan Graphics. Thanks to my editor at McGraw-Hill, Tom Miller.

I'm lucky to have the support of my entire family, especially my "in house" editor, my wife Linda. I would also like to remember my parents, who always supported all my efforts and would have been pleased to see me involved in an educational project like this.

⬦ Contents ⬦

PART THREE
Asthma in Special Circumstances

PART FOUR
Asthma Out of Control

PART FIVE
Special Problems

PART SIX
Conclusion

Appendices

◇ List of Illustrations ◇

xiii

◇ Foreword ◇

One in five Americans suffers from an allergic disease—imagine a disease afflicting nearly fifty million Americans! As such, asthma and allergies are the most common chronic diseases in this country, cause the greatest number of school and work days lost, affect the lives of countless sufferers and their relatives and cost a staggering amount of money. From the perspective of importance of these diseases to the populace, one would anticipate that the medical community would know all aspects of such important diseases. But alas, such is not the case.

Allergies and asthma are chronic, bothersome diseases which (fortunately) are seldom life threatening. Our medical schools tend to focus upon more dangerous and more exotic diseases than allergy, and many of our finest schools do not even have an allergy program or fail to adequately teach the principles and practice of allergy to students and residents. The National Institutes of Health invites a select number of our finest medical students to rotate through our facility each year. During their stay, I provide a lecture on the basic mechanisms of allergy and asthma. Over the past decade I have consistently observed that despite the outstanding record of these students and the repute of their medical schools, they know and understand very little about allergies and asthma. In fact, my lecture is often the only teaching on allergy that these students receive during the clinical phase of their training.

Other than expressing criticism at the adequacy of our medical school curricula, this specific deficiency means that patients and their families cannot rely on their family physician to provide accurate or current information regarding allergy or asthma. To whom then can the allergy or asthma sufferer turn for such advice? The logical answer is the allergist practicing in their community, and he is undoubtedly better equipped to provide such information than anyone else, particularly if he is certified as a diplomate of the American Board of Allergy and Immunology.

There has been an explosion of information about asthma and allergies over the past twenty years. Only practitioners with a commitment to excellence in asthma and allergy are likely to be knowledgeable about current concepts and their application to these diseases. However, the capacity of even the most committed practitioner is limited by the availability of his time and access to concise, accurate literature written for the sufferer. In preparing to write this foreword, I spent time browsing through the shelves devoted to medicine in our local libraries and bookstores. I was impressed with the large number of books written for the allergy sufferer. However, I was shocked and depressed at the inaccurate, misleading, and controversial qualities of many of these books, which were written by medical or paramedical authors expounding claims that are largely unproved by standard scientific methods or even considered to be inappropriate medical practices by our professional organizations. Such books often claimed miracles or new breakthroughs that, if accurate, would better be popularized through scientific proof and medical application rather than through the popular press.

Asthma: The Complete Guide to Self-Management of Asthma and Allergies for Patients and Their Families is a striking and welcome contrast to such books. This readable book was written by a well-trained practitioner who maintains his academic associations, keeps up with advances in the field, and is committed to maintaining a high standard of medical care based upon application of current understanding of the disease process. Asthma and allergic diseases are described clearly, understandably, and accurately. Dr. Weinstein's approach to these diseases and their treatment is based upon years of practice and teaching and the need to better inform sufferers and their families in order to improve therapy.

This book is written for asthma and allergy sufferers, their families, and even for practitioners who wish to learn the facts about these diseases. Moreover, the therapies developed for this book are based upon experience and logic. The therapeutic plans provided should prove useful to both patients and practitioners while the book provides a readable summary of the base of knowledge that is the core to understanding these immensely important diseases.

After carefully reading *Asthma*, I was honored and excited about writing this foreword in order to acclaim this book as an essential part of every asthma and allergy sufferer's library.

MICHAEL KALINER, M.D.
Head, Allergic Diseases Section
National Institute of Allergy and Infectious Diseases
National Institutes of Health
Bethesda, Maryland

◇ Introduction ◇

This book is a practical self-help guide for the estimated eleven million asthma victims in the United States. Asthma sufferers are aware that attacks can occur at any time. This uncertainty makes people with asthma eager for practical self-help techniques for coping with asthma on a daily basis. This book is uniquely designed to fill this need and is a complete and easy-to-use reference package for asthma sufferers.

Asthma is one of the leading causes of missed school and work days in the United States. Over $1 billion is spent each year by asthma sufferers on hospital care, medications, and doctor visits. Studies show that there are twenty-seven million doctor visits annually for treatment of asthma, and over one million of those are first visits. One survey revealed that over 50 percent of asthma patients spend greater than 18 percent of their family income on asthma care.

But the impact of asthma is not merely economic. When asthma symptoms and emergencies occur on a frequent basis—when one must take daily medications and put up with the fatigue, inconvenience, and misconceptions associated with asthma—the impact on the individual and the family can be staggering.

In my private practice I am constantly asked questions by asthma patients and their families that show they want a greater understanding of their illness. And urgent questions arise when asthma patients suffer critical or seemingly critical attacks. These repeated inquiries reflect the frustrations resulting from the asthma sufferer's inability to identify and manage his symptoms.

This book will provide the reader with a clear understanding of the nature of his illness and then provide him with specific techniques to tailor a self-management plan, using his physician's guidance, to monitor and deal effectively with his condition. I believe that the method of dealing with asthma presented in this book will reduce the need for frequent emergency hospital and doctor visits. Ultimately, the asthma sufferer's life will become more orderly and, to a much larger extent, within his own control.

The medication program is the core of this book. If you have limited time, you might want to consider focusing on the first two parts of the book, which provide a basic understanding of asthma and a plan for its treatment. I have provided summaries at the end of each chapter for quick and easy-to-read references. In addition, subheadings are used throughout to highlight topics and organize the information. Questions that are frequently asked by patients and their families are presented with the core material to reinforce the essential points.

Asthma cannot be cured but it can be well managed. Successful self-management requires education. The few brochures and books that have been printed about asthma do not provide sufficiently specific information to accomplish this goal. This book provides the asthma sufferer with the necessary tools for overcoming the fear, confusion, and helplessness often associated with this chronic illness.

PART ONE

❖❖❖❖❖

Understanding
Asthma

❖ 1 ❖

What Is Asthma?

Asthma is best described as obstruction or blockage of the airways (breathing tubes) that is reversible either spontaneously or with proper medication. As the airways narrow, breathing becomes more difficult and a wheezing sound or cough occurs, the result of trying to force air through these blocked air tubes. To best understand how this happens, it is helpful to review the structure of the lung.

Normal Breathing Process. Looking at Figure 1–1, we see that air we breathe in via the nose and mouth passes through the windpipe (trachea), then goes into two large air tubes (bronchi), one for each lung. These large air tubes divide like the branches of a tree, within the lung itself, into small air tubes (bronchioles) which lead to air sacs (alveoli). It is in the air sacs that an important exchange occurs: The oxygen that we breathe in is transferred to the blood (via small blood vessels called capillaries) for the body's work, and carbon dioxide, the waste product of the body's work, is returned to the air sacs and exhaled. Figure 1–2 shows the constriction of the airways that occurs during an asthma flare.

Asthma Versus Emphysema. Asthma affects only the air tubes, not the air sacs. The diagnosis of emphysema (rather

Normal Breathing Process

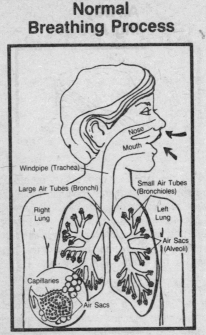

Air is taken in through the nose and mouth and passes through the windpipe (trachea) and into the lungs through the two large air tubes (bronchi). Air then passes into the small air tubes (bronchioles) and into the air sacs (alveoli). In the air sacs, oxygen is transferred into the blood via the small blood vessels called capillaries, and carbon dioxide is returned to the air sacs and exhaled.

Figure 1–1

than asthma) is made when the walls of the air sacs are damaged or destroyed and the exchange of oxygen and carbon dioxide into the blood is impaired. The most common cause of emphysema is cigarette smoking; there are some rare con-

Airways During Asthma

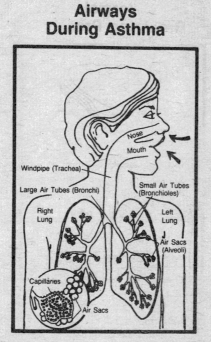

Asthma affects the air tubes, not the air sacs. With asthma symptoms the air tubes become narrow, making it difficult for air to move through the lungs.

Figure 1-2

genital causes in nonsmokers. It is important to emphasize that because asthma affects the air tubes but not the air sacs, and because asthma is a reversible process, it does not lead to emphysema.

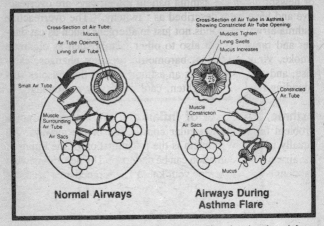

During an asthma flare, the muscles surrounding the air tubes tighten.
There is inflammation and swelling of the air tube lining. There is also
an increase in mucus which clogs the air tubes. This is why it is so
difficult to breathe during an asthma attack.

Figure 1–3

Factors That Cause Asthma. Figure 1–3 describes the
three factors that can cause the airways to become narrowed
and blocked during an asthma flare: (1) constriction of the
muscles surrounding the air tubes, (2) inflammation and
swelling of the lining of the air tubes, and (3) increased mucus production that clogs the air tubes.

Muscular Constriction: "Twitchy" Airways. The air
tube is made up of several layers. On the outside of the air
tube there is muscle which, by tightening and relaxing, controls the size of the opening of the air tube (the space through
which air must pass). The muscle works by reflex, and is
guided by the same portions of the nervous system that control reflexes such as involuntary blinking. We have little con-
scious control over the tightening and relaxing of these
muscles. Everyone's airways have the potential for constricting in response to irritants such as cigarette smoke, perfume,

or newsprint. In the asthma patient the airways are overreactive and have been described as "twitchy." The overreactive asthma airway responds not just to allergens (such as cat dander and ragweed) but also to other factors such as cigarette smoke, viral infections, barometric pressure changes, exercise, and cold air. During an asthma attack, the muscles surrounding the airways tighten, causing airway narrowing.

Asthma, a Disease of Inflammation. Asthma is not a problem limited to muscular constriction of the airways. An equally important problem is the inflammation of the lining of the airways. Inflammation can be understood by describing what happens when you scrape your knee. The scraped area becomes swollen and oozes with a fluid that contains many kinds of cells, some of which help to fight infection. However, this fluid also contributes to the swelling. In asthma, the innermost lining of the airways is filled with cells and fluid that, as with the scraped knee, are a product of the inflammatory response. These cells and the associated swelling contribute to the obstruction of the airways in asthma. Steroids, the medication most often utilized for difficult-to-manage flares of asthma, help to reduce inflammation in the airways.

Mucus Plugs. Mucus, which normally lubricates the airways to allow air to flow smoothly, increases in amount during asthma flares and serves as a sticky plug to clog the airways, especially the smaller ones. All asthma patients are aware of the sensation of trying to cough up mucus. Often they feel that if they could clear their airways by coughing up a sufficient amount of mucus, their asthma symptoms would subside. But frequently there is so much mucus that even if one mucus plug is brought up, the same sensation and symptoms persist. It is important to seek your doctor's advice early on if you are unable to clear mucus plugging your airways, since neglected mucus plugging often prolongs asthma flares. In addition, when the plugs are allowed to linger they can become a source of infection. For this reason an antibiotic is often prescribed for patients who are slow to respond to treatment when their asthma flares.

Asthma Attacks. Asthma occurs in attacks at varying time intervals. Attacks can be as brief as several minutes or as lengthy as hours or days. Between attacks there may be symptom-free intervals when it is impossible to tell an asthma patient from someone who does not have asthma. A breathing test called spirometry, which is used to determine whether a person has asthma, may be normal in an asthma patient during asthma-free intervals. On the other hand, some people have asthma symptoms continuously, and their spirometry tests reflect this. Still others have subtle asthma symptoms such as a hacking cough or chest tightness. For these symptoms, spirometry is an important clue for determining whether the patient has asthma, and should be part of the doctor's evaluation.

Developing Your Asthma Case History. Table 1–1 leads you through a series of questions that will help you to understand your asthma history so that you can clearly communicate this information to your doctor.

As you can see, asthma symptoms can be quite varied. In addition to wheezing, symptoms can range from a tickle in the throat to a dry cough without wheezing. More typically, patients cough to clear mucus from the airways. For some patients, the extent of mucus production can be a major problem. Coughing triggered by laughter may also be a subtle sign of asthma. Asthma patients also report shortness of breath (only with asthma flares and not on a routine basis unless asthma symptoms are daily), tightness in the chest, and particular trouble exhaling (as opposed to breathing in) as a result of the airway obstruction.

It is important to be aware that not all wheezing is due to asthma. Obstructions of the upper airway such as a foreign body or polyps of the vocal cords can cause symptoms that mimic asthma. Other problems such as heart failure and lung cancer can cause wheezing and be misinterpreted as asthma. It is important to have a chest X-ray as part of your asthma evaluation, since asthma alone does not give rise to an abnormal chest X-ray. (See Chapter 18.)

You must tell your doctor whether your asthma symptoms occur only occasionally or on a daily basis. In addition, the times of day, surroundings, and conditions typically associ-

Developing Your Asthma Case History

Place a checkmark next to the symptoms and descriptions which apply to you.

* Do you have any of the following possible symptoms of asthma:
  — Shortness of breath?
  — Wheezing?
  — Coughing?
  — Coughing along with wheezing?
  — Tickle in the throat leading to coughing?
  — Coughing which produces mucus? Clear mucus? Discolored mucus?
  — Coughing brought on by laughter?
  — Chest tightness?
  — Shortness of breath with physical exertion?

* Do you feel that your wheezing comes from:
  — Your neck? (indicating a possible upper airway blockage)
  — Your chest? (pointing to asthma as the possible cause)

* Do you have asthma symptoms:
  — On a daily basis?
  — Only occasionally?
  — Only under certain conditions? (for example, around animals, in cold weather, with infections)

* Are your symptoms:
  — Worse at night? (see page 277)
  — Worse at work? (see page 232)
  — Worse at home or during weekends?
  — Worse outdoors? (see page 186)
  — Worse indoors?
  — Worse or better in different parts of the country?

* Do your symptoms:
  — Begin suddenly?
  — Gradually become worse over time?
  — Flare only with infections?
  — Vary with the allergy seasons?

Table 1-1

- Do you have upper respiratory problems such as:
  — Sinusitis?
  — Hay fever?
  — Postnasal drip?
  — Nasal polyps? (see page 285)

- Do you have a hiatus hernia, belch repeatedly, or have a sour taste in your mouth after eating? (see page 282)

- Did your asthma become worse during pregnancy?

- Do you have a history of heart problems? (see page 311)

- Are you a cigarette smoker?

- Was your most recent chest X-ray normal? (An abnormal chest X-ray may point to another cause for your wheezing.)

In completing your case history, it is also important to pinpoint which factors precipitate your asthma attacks (see Chapter 2, page 16.)

Table 1-1 (continued)

ated with your asthma symptoms may provide clues to your doctor which will help to determine the best therapy. The pattern of your symptoms is also important for determining the best treatment for your asthma. For example, the approach will vary according to whether symptoms begin suddenly, begin gradually, flare with infection, or vary with the allergy seasons. Consideration should be given to the possibility that an upper respiratory problem (such as sinusitis or nasal polyps) could be a trigger of your asthma symptoms.

In completing your case history, it is also important to pinpoint the factors that precipitate your asthma attacks (see Table 1-2) as well as specific elements in your environment which may play a role in your asthma (Chapter 6).

Asthma Out of Control. During a serious asthma attack, the combination of muscular constriction of the airways, swelling and inflammation of the lining of the airways, and excessive mucus secretion can result in severe airway blockage with little

---

Factors That Can Trigger Asthma Symptoms

1. Infection (usually viral in nature; underlying sinus infection must be considered)

2. Allergens (such as seasonal pollens, dust, mold, animal dander)

3. Exercise

4. Aspirin and tartazine (yellow food dye #5)

5. Emotional upset

6. Irritants (such as cigarette smoke, perfumes, air pollution)

7. Cold air and changes in weather

8. Foods (in rare cases) and food additives such as sulfites

Table 1–2

or no air movement beyond the obstruction. Overinflation of the lungs occurs due to this blockage, as the patient cannot exhale all the air within his lungs normally. This trapped air is stale since its oxygen has already been transported from the air sacs into the bloodstream. Since enough fresh oxygen cannot pass beyond the blockage and into the lungs, the routine exchange of carbon dioxide (the body's waste product) and oxygen can no longer fully take place within the air sacs. Carbon dioxide builds up in the bloodstream while the oxygen content of the blood drops. When this occurs the situation may well be life threatening. It is for this reason that in the emergency room during a severe asthma attack, blood is drawn from the patient's artery to check the blood's oxygen and carbon dioxide content. This information gives the doctor a clearer understanding of the severity of the attack.

The Importance of Early Treatment. Asthma is best treated early to avoid the potentially life-threatening sequence of events described above. If you routinely have asthma flares that require emergency room visits, your management program should be reevaluated with your doctor so that a more satisfactory result can be achieved. Keep your doctor informed of your progress. Asthma management programs often cannot be perfected the first time you visit your doctor. Modifications may be necessary since response to medication varies from patient to patient.

Asthma symptoms are relieved by bronchodilators (medicine to open the airways) or, if symptoms are severe, by steroids, to reduce inflammation. Emphasis is also placed on helping the patient to clear any mucus plugs. An overview of the available medications and techniques utilized in asthma management will be presented so that you will better understand your asthma and the plan outlined by your doctor. A carefully designed asthma plan will assure that you are prepared to treat your symptoms early, before they get out of control, even if asthma symptoms occur suddenly. This approach will ultimately give you the confidence and reassurance necessary to limit the impact of asthma on your life.

QUESTIONS

1. How do I know if I have asthma?

Clues that indicate that you might have asthma include a history of wheezing, coughing, or chest tightness, often accompanied by shortness of breath. These symptoms tend to recur in certain situations such as when you are around cats, when you exercise, or when you have an infection. You should see a doctor, who will review your history, listen to your chest, and have you perform a breathing test called spirometry. This test compares your ability to expel air forcefully with the ability of people without asthma of your same age and height. If your breathing test result is below normal this might be an indication that you have asthma, since the asthma sufferer must breathe out through blocked airways. The doctor will then give you two puffs of an asthma inhaler. If your airways open even partially in response to the inhaled medication, the diagnosis of asthma can be made, since the criterion of asthma as *reversible* obstructive airway disease has been met.

2. If I don't wheeze, can I have asthma?

Possibly. Blockage of the airway can be quite subtle or quite dramatic. Symptoms of asthma can run the full range from mild shortness of breath without coughing or wheezing, to flagrant shortness of breath without wheezing (because there is so little air movement that there is no wheezing sound). Symptoms that fall between these extremes, such as coughing along with wheezing, are more typical.

3. If I have asthma, can I also have emphysema?

Yes. Smoking is the primary cause of emphysema. Smokers with asthma run the same or greater risk of developing emphysema as smokers who do not have asthma. The most simple solution is not to smoke, especially in light of all the evidence today of the health risks of cigarette smoking. The damage to the air sacs caused by emphysema is *irreversible*, because with emphysema the walls between the air sacs are permanently broken down. As a result, there is less surface area for the exchange of oxygen and carbon dioxide to occur. Less oxygen passes into the circulation, causing a build-up in the bloodstream of the body's waste product, carbon dioxide. Patients with emphysema are often short of breath and unable to exert themselves. Emphysema often leads to progressive severe disability and the routine need for supplemental oxygen.

If you are worried that you might have emphysema, check with your doctor. Clues that the doctor uses in making the diagnosis of emphysema include: (a) routine shortness of breath with moderate physical exertion (such as walking briskly or up stairs); (b) long history of cigarette smoking; (c) physical examination which reveals findings such as faint breath sounds when listening to the chest, indicating that too much air remains in the chest as a result of the breakdown of the air sacs; and (d) laboratory studies such as a chest X-ray, breathing tests including spirometry and a diffusion capacity of the lung for carbon monoxide study (DLCO), and a study to determine the amount of oxygen in the arterial blood after exercise. Since the air sacs are damaged with emphysema and oxygen is not transferred to the blood as effectively, it is easy to understand that the oxygen content in the arterial blood in a person with emphysema would be reduced, especially with exercise. The diagnosis of emphysema is confirmed by a diffusion study, which implies that the diffusion of oxygen from the air sacs is impaired.

4. If I suffer frequently from bronchitis, could I have asthma?

Yes. People who have bronchitis (inflammation of the air tubes accompanied by coughing and mucus) may well have underlying asthma. Often the diagnosis of asthma in this setting is confirmed by spirometry. If this is the case, treatment of your bronchitis may be helped by adding asthma medications.

5. My asthma occurs only in the spring. Will my symptoms get worse?

There is no way of predicting. Asthma runs a variable course—it can occur at any age and can subside at any time. For most people, asthma will follow a pattern. If you have allergies to tree or grass pollen in the spring, your asthma symptoms will probably get worse each spring as the pollen count rises. Asthma symptoms can often be anticipated on the basis of your history and appropriate preparatory measures can be taken.

6. I hear wheezing from my throat, not from my chest. I take asthma medications but they don't seem to help. What should I do?

This is an important observation which should be brought to your doctor's attention. Consultation with an otolaryngologist (ear, nose, and throat doctor) is in order to obtain a careful examination of your upper airway. Examples of upper airway problems which could be causing your wheezing include the presence of foreign bodies (such as a coin or a food particle), growths in the windpipe and vocal cords, and congenital problems (such as weakness of the cartilage of the windpipe). Upper airway problems can often be long-standing and sometimes cause symptoms that can be confused with asthma symptoms.

7. I am sixty-five years old and just recently developed asthma. How is this possible?

It is possible to develop asthma at any age, but it is essential for you to have a careful examination to exclude the possibility of an underlying problem such as subtle heart failure, called cardiac asthma (page 311). A chest X-ray is helpful as it may reveal enlargement of the heart, which is present with cardiac asthma; the chest X-ray with asthma is usually normal in appearance.

SUMMARY: WHAT IS ASTHMA?

1. Asthma is best described as reversible obstructive airway disease.

2. The obstruction (blockage) of the airways (breathing tubes) occurs as a result of: (a) tightening of the muscles surrounding the airways; (b) swelling and inflammation of the lining of the air tubes; and (c) increased mucus production. The blockage can be reversed with proper medications.

3. The airways of an asthma sufferer are overreactive and ready to respond to various stimuli.

4. Asthma affects the airways, not the air sacs, and is reversible. Therefore asthma does not lead to emphysema, which causes permanent damage to the air sac walls.

5. Asthma is a chronic, long-term illness that can occur at any time. Asthma typically occurs in attacks spaced with symptom-free intervals, but it may also occur on a continuous basis.

6. Asthma symptoms can vary and are not limited to wheezing. For example, a subtle cough, without wheezing, can be the sole symptom of asthma. Furthermore, it is important to be aware that not all wheezing is due to asthma. Table 1-1 (page 9) helps you to develop your own asthma case history.

♦ 2 ♦

Factors That Can Trigger Asthma Symptoms

Asthma has been analogized with a cocked gun. An asthma attack can be triggered at any time by various familiar and unfamiliar precipitating factors. Table 2–1 lists the major factors that can precipitate asthma symptoms. The typical asthma patient is affected by a combination of these factors, each of which will be discussed below. As you read each section, refer to the checklist (Table 2–1) to help you summarize which factors trigger your symptoms.

A. ALLERGIES

Not everyone who has asthma is allergic. However, allergy can without question play a role in asthma symptoms for some individuals. The pattern and timing of the patient's asthma symptoms often provide clues suggesting that allergy may be causing the asthma. Seasonal pollens from trees and grasses in the spring and ragweed in the fall can precipitate an asthma episode during those times of the year. Exposure to dog or cat dander, feather pillows, dust, and molds can all precipitate year-round symptoms.

The mechanism whereby allergens can cause nasal and asthma symptoms is shown in Figure 2–1. There is a cell

Checklist:
What Factors Trigger Your Asthma Symptoms?

☐ **Allergy**   Notes
   — Seasonal symptoms?
      Spring—trees, grasses
      Fall—ragweed   _____
   — Year-round symptoms?
      Dust, mold, animal dander,
      feathers   _____

☐ **Infection**
   — Colds?   _____
   — Sinus infections?   _____

                                          _____
☐ **Aspirin and Aspirin-Containing
   Products**
   — Cross-reacting medications?
      (See Table 2–4)   _____
   — Tartrazine (yellow food dye
      # 5)?   _____

☐ **Exercise**   _____
   — Asthma worse with
      _____?   _____
      (Type of exercise)
   — Asthma worse with cold air?   _____

☐ **Irritants**   _____
   — Cigarette smoke?
   — Perfume?   _____
   — Newsprint?
   — Hairspray?   _____
   — Deodorant?
   — Household cleaners?   _____

                                          _____
☐ **Foods**
   — Sulfites?
   — Wheat, milk, nuts, other   _____
      _____?   _____

Table 2–1

☐ **Emotional Upset**   Notes
   — Asthma worse with personal
     tension and stress?
   _____

☐ **Weather Conditions**   _____
   — Air pollution?
   — Cold air?   _____
   — Rapid temperature changes?

☐ **Miscellaneous**   _____
   — Occupational exposure? (Chapter
     10)   _____
   — Pregnancy? (Chapter 9)
   — Nighttime asthma? (Chapter 15)   _____
   — Gastroesophageal reflux? (Chap-
     ter 16)   _____

Table 2–1 (continued)

called the mast cell which is found throughout the body, including the nose, the airways, and the skin. Attached to the
mast cell in allergic individuals is an antibody called IgE.
This is the antibody which is typically involved with allergy.
This antibody develops with repeated exposure to the particular allergen over a period of time. One usually thinks of
antibodies as the body's defense system for fighting infection.
However, in an allergic individual, the body's defense system
responds to allergens in the environment such as dust, pollen,
or animal dander.

There is a specific IgE antibody for each allergen to which
you are sensitive. For example, if you are allergic to ragweed,
you have the IgE antibody to ragweed sitting on the mast
cells in your body. Many IgE antibodies to different allergens
can sit on a single mast cell. A mast cell can accommodate
several hundred thousand IgE antibodies. When the IgE antibody sitting on the mast cell is exposed to the allergen to
which it reacts, chemicals called mediators are released from

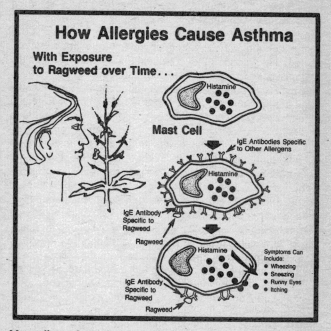

Mast cells are found throughout the body, including the nose, the airways, and the skin. With exposure over time to an allergen (such as ragweed), an allergic individual produces antibodies (called IgE) to the specific type of allergen. IgE antibodies sit on the mast cells in the nose and airways. When the person is exposed to ragweed, the ragweed allergen attaches to the IgE for ragweed sitting on the mast cell. Histamine is then released from the mast cell, which causes various allergic symptoms and can trigger an asthma flare.

Figure 2–1

the mast cell. These chemical mediators cause you to experience various allergic responses. The most common chemical mediator is histamine, which can cause nasal runniness and stuffiness, as well as itchy, watery eyes typical of hay fever, and asthma symptoms.

Other chemical mediators released from the mast cells include the leukotrienes and the prostaglandins. The leukotrienes are of particular importance in asthma research because they seem to cause sustained constriction of the muscles of the airways. Although there are several medications to counter some of the effects of mast cell mediator release, there is no agent currently available to block the effect of the leukotrienes. There is extensive research taking place in this regard. Some prostaglandins have the ability to open the airways while others are able to constrict the airways. Research is under way to try to develop a new approach to asthma therapy utilizing the prostaglandins that open the airways.

If your medical history points to allergy as a possible trigger of your asthma symptoms, skin testing is an easy way to confirm the diagnosis. If you are allergic, the specific antibody for the allergen to which you are sensitive is already attached to mast cells in your skin. When a small amount of the allergen is placed on or under your skin during an allergy skin test, the IgE antibody is exposed to the allergen, resulting in mast cell release of chemical mediators into the skin. The mediators cause a reaction in the skin, the raised area of which is called a wheal and the red area a flare. If you are not allergic to the specific allergen that was placed on or under your skin, there will be no reaction or only a very slight reaction in the skin.

The best way of managing allergy is to avoid the offending allergen (although this is not always possible). Therefore, it is probably not wise for an asthma patient with an allergic tendency to have a cat or a dog as a pet. There is the risk that with time, allergy to the pet will develop and asthma symptoms will become more frequent due to routine exposure to the pet. Without question, the most effective treatment for an allergy to animal dander is to give the pet away. Although this may be a difficult step to take, it may be necessary if you notice that your asthma symptoms disappear when you are away from your pet. If giving up the pet is impossible, a logical next step is to limit the pet's access to the bedroom. The bedroom should be an allergy patient's haven.

The bedroom door should remain closed to prevent the pet from entering the room even if you are not at home.

The seasonal pollens are more difficult to avoid because they are airborne and so small that they cannot be seen. The most practical suggestions for the seasonal pollens include keeping your bedroom and car windows closed to prevent airborne pollens from entering, and using air conditioning instead. A more extensive discussion of steps you can take to reduce your allergic exposure is presented in Chapter 6.

If you feel that allergies may contribute to your asthma symptoms, ask your doctor to refer you to an allergist certified by the American Board of Allergy and Clinical Immunology for a diagnostic evaluation including allergy skin testing. With the allergist's help you can work out a plan for avoiding the things to which you are allergic and for taking medications to manage your allergy/asthma symptoms. Allergy shots (immunotherapy) can also be considered if your medical history and allergy skin test results suggest that they may be of benefit. A more detailed approach to allergies is found in Chapter 17.

QUESTIONS

1. What is the difference between allergies and asthma?

Asthma is blockage of the airways that can be reversed. Allergies are one of the factors that can trigger asthma symptoms in a person with asthma. Allergies develop over time in someone who is born with a tendency to develop allergies. On reexposure to the substance to which one is allergic (the allergen), symptoms can result that can involve the nose (hay fever), the eyes (allergic conjunctivitis), the skin (hives and eczema), as well as the airways (asthma). Therefore, the airways are just one of the parts of the body that can be involved with allergies.

2. I have hay fever during the ragweed season. Although my symptoms involve only my nose, am I likely to develop asthma in subsequent years?

There is no way of predicting. A percentage of people who

have hay fever will develop asthma, but most will not. To date there are no routine tests that can predict which individuals with allergies are likely to develop asthma. There is no reason to assume that you will develop asthma simply because your allergies are left untreated. If allergy shots are necessary for your hay fever, it should be kept in mind that the reason for the injections is to manage your nasal symptoms, not to prevent asthma.

3. It seems as if I have allergies year round but am worse in the spring. What could be the cause of my allergies?

House dust, molds, feathers, and animal dander are the classic allergens that trigger year-round symptoms. Irritants such as cigarette smoke, hair sprays, and perfumes can all mimic allergens. Spring allergies are usually due to tree pollen or mold spores in the early spring, and grass pollen in the late spring and early summer. Weeds such as English plaintain can also cause springtime allergy symptoms. Ragweed, some other weeds, and mold spores all contribute to symptoms in the latter part of summer and early fall. This pattern can vary in different parts of the country (see page 341 to determine the seasonal pattern for your area). An allergist can confirm your allergic history by performing allergy skin testing. If allergies seem to play a role in your asthma, it is wise to seek the opinion of an allergist who has been certified by the American Board of Allergy and Clinical Immunology.

4. During a visit to a different part of the country, I noticed that my asthma and hay fever symptoms improved dramatically. If I move there, is this change likely to be permanent?

It is impossible to predict whether your asthma symptoms would eventually return. If your asthma is triggered by factors such as air pollution or a cold climate, then a move to a different geographical area could possibly bring about a long-lasting improvement in your symptoms. If your asthma is triggered by allergies, however, a move to a new area may bring about only a temporary improvement in asthma symptoms, since you may develop new allergies in subsequent years as you become exposed to different allergens. It is for this reason that allergists usually do not recommend that a patient move to another part of the country without first trying an extended visit to the new area and without first warning the patient that asthma symptoms may return. You should discuss your thoughts carefully with your doctor. Generally, moves to another part of the country do not improve asthma and allergies in the long run, and are often accompanied by great financial and personal hardship for the entire family.

5. Every time my child sees her allergist, the nurse gives me a sheet of paper with instructions concerning dust avoidance. These suggestions would require major modifications in my pattern of living. Is it worth the effort it would take to carry out these suggestions?

If you notice that your child has increased asthma symptoms when exposed to dust and this has been confirmed by your allergist, it is wise to follow environmental precautions with regard to dust. Certainly the first step is to make your child's bedroom as free of dust as possible, as she probably sleeps at least eight hours in that room each night (see page 190 concerning dust control measures). Studies have shown that attention to environmental allergens can greatly reduce asthma symptoms and the need for medication. Therefore, your doctor's suggestions concerning dust avoidance are worth the effort.

SUMMARY: ALLERGY

1. Allergies can trigger an asthma attack in an allergic individual who has asthma. Not everyone who has asthma is allergic.

2. Allergies develop with repeated exposure to an allergen. It takes time to develop allergies.

3. Allergies are best managed by: (a) avoidance of the offending allergen if possible; (b) judicious use of medications to manage allergy symptoms; and (c) allergy shots to reduce your sensitivity to the allergen. If you are allergic, an allergist is an important part of your asthma-management team.

B. INFECTIONS

Infections can be caused by bacteria, viruses, and fungi (molds). Bacterial infections include strep throat and some pneumonias, while the most frequent viral infection is the common cold. Bacterial infections respond to treatment with antibiotics; viral infections do not.

Infections, especially viral infections, can lead to a flare of asthma symptoms. It is not unusual for a cold to trigger or eventually lead to wheezing or coughing. It has been observed that asthma patients are more susceptible to upper respiratory infections; however, the explanation for this is not clear-cut. One possible factor may be the increased mucus typically present in the upper airway of an asthma patient. Certain other viruses, such as flu virus, can also trigger increased airway irritability and lead to an asthma attack.

Bacterial infections such as strep throat or pneumonias of bacterial origin can also be associated with asthma flares. However, these infections do not cause asthma to flare with the same frequency as do viral infections. Oftentimes bacterial infections occur as a complication of an asthma attack, especially if it has taken several days to bring the attack fully under control. In all probability, the mucus plugging the airway or the area of the lung behind the mucus plug becomes infected because the mucus cannot be coughed up and cleared.

Asthma symptoms sometimes first develop shortly after an infection such as bronchitis or pneumonia. This is referred to as postpneumonic or postbronchitic bronchospasm. In this situation asthma symptoms persist for a variable time period, from a few weeks to several months, although in some individuals asthma symptoms persist on a more permanent basis.

A prevailing viewpoint among doctors is that if children wheeze only as a result of infections, and do not have asthma flares from other causes such as allergies, the likelihood is greater that they will not have asthma in later years.

Since asthma attacks can come on quite suddenly and dramatically, it is best to be prepared with an asthma medication program that can be initiated early. It is important to be a step ahead to avoid the need for an emergency room visit. In addition, if the mucus from your nose or chest is yellowish or greenish in color, this may indicate that you have an infection; notify your doctor so that he can prescribe an antibiotic for you. Also, congestion in the upper airways (the nose, sinuses, and throat) often has a negative effect on the lower airways (the breathing tubes). Treatment of upper airway congestion often leads to an improvement in asthma symptoms.

Flu and pneumococcal pneumonia vaccinations are available as preventative measures, and asthma is one of the indications for their use. Flu vaccinations only prevent the strain of virus which is expected to cause flu symptoms that year; they do not prevent colds. Check with your doctor to see if you are a candidate for these shots.

Sinus infections (sinusitis), which at times can be quite subtle and chronic, can also make asthma symptoms worse. An X-ray examination of the sinuses may be necessary to determine whether they are infected. Certainly any asthma patient who is experiencing the classic symptoms of sinusitis should be treated. Typical symptoms of sinusitis include headache over the affected sinus area, achiness radiating to the teeth, pressure over the cheeks or forehead, nausea, and yellowish or greenish discharge from the nose. In addition, there can also be postnasal drip and a slightly sore throat as a result of the nasal drainage. Fever is also possible but may be absent. In those individuals affected by sinusitis in association with asthma, identification and management of the underlying sinus problem may well be the essential key to better asthma management.

QUESTIONS

1. My nose is always stuffy. How can I tell whether it is from an infection (such as a cold) or from allergy?

Sometimes it is difficult to distinguish a cold from routine allergy symptoms. Clues that tend to indicate that you have an infection include fever, a scratchy or sore throat, achiness, chills, and a change in mucus color. If you think you might have an infection and your asthma symptoms are affected, notify your doctor. Your doctor may want to culture your throat to rule out strep throat, or to draw blood to look for clues in your white blood cell count that might distinguish an infection from allergy. An antibiotic will not help you if you have a viral infection such as a cold. Antibiotics simply do not work against viruses. However, an antibiotic may be helpful to prevent complications of an infection, such as a bacterial infection that can't be cleared from blocked airways during prolonged asthma symptoms.

2. Lots of people have sinus congestion. Why is it so important?

If you have asthma, it is very important for your doctor to know about and treat any sinus problems you may have. Underlying infections such as sinusitis can be a constant trigger for asthma symptoms. Doctors today understand that problems in the upper airways (the sinuses and the nose) can have impact on the lower airways in the chest and trigger wheezing or coughing. You can help your doctor provide you with better care by pointing out any history of sinus problems. (See Chapter 17.)

3. I take asthma medications every day. If I get an infection, should I take more asthma medicine or just start taking an antibiotic?

Every asthma medication has a dosage that is appropriate for you. Do not take any extra medication without your doctor's permission. If you find that your routine medications are not sufficient in this situation, review with your doctor a backup choice. Don't just take extra medications on your own.

In addition, don't start taking an antibiotic without your doctor's knowledge, as the antibiotic may hide an infection that would be important to identify, possibly with a culture. A culture provides the doctor with the specific name of the bacteria that is causing your infection, so that the appropriate treatment course can be prescribed. If you start the antibiotic before the culture is taken, it may be impossible to make the proper diagnosis. However, there are exceptions to this rule. For some patients, the value of starting the antibiotic early may outweigh the information that can be obtained with a culture. The right approach for you must be worked out with your doctor. Once the antibiotic is started, you must fully complete the prescribed course.

In addition, use of the antibiotic erythromycin causes the blood theophylline level to rise. If this antibiotic is used, an appropriate reduction in your dose of theophylline should be made, typically by 20 percent. Finally, be sure that any antibiotic that you use is fresh, as old antibiotics can lead to serious problems such as kidney damage. If there is any question in this regard, ask your pharmacist or your doctor.

SUMMARY: INFECTIONS

1. Viral infections such as colds are the most common infections that lead to asthma flares.

2. Although bacterial infections such as strep throat can in rare cases be the cause of an asthma attack, it is more likely for a bacterial infection to occur as a result of a difficult asthma attack, when mucus which can't be cleared because of blocked airways eventually becomes infected.

3. As asthma symptoms can begin suddenly, it is important to be prepared with your asthma plan and to start it early.

4. Notify your doctor early if any yellowish or greenish mucus is coming from your nose or from your chest, or if your asthma medication plan does not seem to be controlling your symptoms.

5. Check with your doctor to see if you are a candidate for either the current flu vaccine or the pneumococcal pneumonia vaccine.

6. Underlying sinus problems can be a constant trigger for asthma symptoms. Notify your doctor if you experience sinus symptoms.

C. EXERCISE

A common misconception among parents, asthma sufferers, and even some doctors is that people with asthma cannot exercise at all or can only engage in minimal exercise. However, with rare exception, asthma patients can fully participate in exercise programs if they understand the mechanism by which exercise induces an asthma attack, and use pretreatment techniques to avoid such attacks.

Exercise triggers asthma symptoms under specific conditions. Strenuous, continuous exercise causes rapid breathing through the mouth. As a result, the air that reaches the air tubes has not been warmed and humidified by the nose and upper airway as it usually is with routine normal breathing through the nose. The rapid introduction of cold, dry air into the air tubes has been shown to trigger the asthma response.

This helps to explain why certain sports are more likely than others to cause asthma symptoms. For example, swimming causes less asthma symptoms than jogging. While swimming, you inhale air from just above the waterline. Since this air is humid even though it enters the air tubes directly from the mouth, the asthma response is less likely to occur. A different situation occurs with jogging. As you begin to breathe rapidly through the mouth while jogging, the air reaching the breathing tubes is not warmed and humidified in the usual manner. Drying of the airways occurs, leading to asthma symptoms in some individuals. Jogging during the winter can be particularly difficult since the air that reaches your airways is not only dry but cold as well. The use of a face mask or scarf over your mouth while exercising in cold air can often be helpful.

Treadmill running under laboratory conditions has shown that asthma symptoms are most likely to occur within six to eight minutes after exercise begins. For most asthma patients, running less than six minutes actually opens the airways. Running longer than six minutes allows some asthma patients to "run through" their symptoms. This confirms observations often mentioned by patients, but does not suggest that asthma patients should keep exercising until they are able to "run through" their asthma. If exercise is stopped due to asthma symptoms, the symptoms usually subside on their own over the next few minutes to one hour. If this is not the case, you should use your back-up medication and notify your doctor.

In view of these observations, it makes sense for asthma patients to choose a sport that does not require continuous exercise, such as baseball, football, golf, or tennis, as opposed to a sustained activity such as cross-country skiing or long-distance running. Swimming is thought to be the best exercise for patients with exercise-induced asthma. However, proper conditioning along with a carefully worked-out regimen for pretreatment prior to exercise often allows asthma patients to participate in any type of exercise. Proper warm-up prior to strenuous exercise is important, and may be helpful for avoiding symptoms during the critical time period when asthma symptoms are most likely to occur during exercise. Practical suggestions for exercise-induced asthma are listed in Table 2–2. Medication management of exercise-induced asthma is reviewed in Chapter 5.

QUESTIONS

1. Every time I start to run I have to stop because of coughing and chest tightness from my asthma. Will I ever be able to exercise?

If your problem is solely related to asthma, then you probably will be able to exercise. The first step is to see your asthma doctor to review your previous experiences during exercise and to have a physical examination and a breathing test. The breathing test, measured by a spirometer, indicates whether your routine lung function is less than it should be. If this is the case, the use of asthma medication on a daily basis along with a pretreatment medication prior to exercise may be necessary to block the exercise-induced asthma response. If your breathing test is normal, medication used prior to exercise is by itself usually sufficient to block exercise-induced asthma, without the need for daily medications. The most common pretreatment medications are inhaled medica-

Suggestions for Exercise-Induced Asthma

- Choose a sport that does not require sustained exercise, such as baseball, golf, or weight lifting, rather than a continuous activity such as long-distance running or aerobic dancing.

- Try to avoid exercise which takes place in cold, dry environments, such as ice skating and cross-country skiing. Swimming is considered to be the best sport for a person with exercise-induced asthma.

- If you must exercise in the cold, try using a face mask or scarf over your mouth and nose to warm and humidify the air you breathe.

- Use a warm-up period to try to avoid asthma symptoms which typically occur during the first fifteen minutes of exercise.

- Develop a preexercise medication plan with your doctor to try to block exercise-induced asthma (see Chapter 5). If your asthma flares despite pretreatment, have a back-up medication plan ready to use if symptoms persist after stopping exercise.

Table 2–2

tions such as albuterol (Proventil or Ventolin), metaproterenol (Alupent or Metaprel), and cromolyn sodium (Intal). See page 158 for suggested medication programs for exercise-induced asthma; your specific program should be designed by your doctor. Without question, you should choose a form of exercise that is reasonable in view of your lung status and level of physical condition.

2. When I start to wheeze during exercise, I use my inhaler. It usually helps but my exercise is interrupted. What should I do?

If you routinely develop asthma symptoms during exercise, you should routinely use your preexercise regimen. Questions do arise when exercise-induced asthma symptoms occur only sporadically. It then becomes a personal decision, made with your doctor's help, whether to use your preexercise regimen every time you exercise. This is an important decision because inhaled medications are effective in blocking exercise-induced asthma only if taken before exercise begins.

SUMMARY: EXERCISE

1. Exercise can trigger asthma symptoms in some individuals, but this does not mean that people with asthma should not or cannot exercise.

2. Exercise-induced asthma usually follows a pattern, with symptoms typically reaching their peak after six to eight minutes of continuous, strenuous exercise. Asthma symptoms usually subside without need for treatment within several minutes but can linger up to one hour. If symptoms persist longer than a few minutes after stopping exercise, you should turn to your back-up medication program.

3. Asthma is thought to occur during exercise when rapid breathing (usually through the mouth) introduces cold, nonhumidified air into the airways, triggering an asthma response. Normally, air is warmed and humidified in the nose and upper airways before it passes into the lower airways.

4. Swimming is considered to be the exercise least likely to bring on asthma symptoms.

5. Use of a pretreatment regimen and back-up medication plan prepared by the patient's doctor, as well as proper conditioning with a warm-up period prior to exercise, should allow most asthma patients to participate fully in the exercise of their choice without developing asthma symptoms.

D. ASPIRIN AND TARTRAZINE (YELLOW FOOD DYE #5)

Aspirin and products that contain aspirin can trigger asthma attacks in certain individuals. The attacks can begin with little warning and can be severe. In addition to causing rapid onset attacks, aspirin can also cause asthma to be more difficult to manage in certain patients who have routine asthma symptoms.

This response to aspirin is not an allergic reaction, as there is no IgE "allergy" antibody directed to aspirin. However, the exact mechanism for this reaction is not clear-cut. It has been termed an idiosyncratic or unanticipated reaction. Studies show that as many as one in every five to ten asthma patients experience a drop in their lung function of at least 20 percent after using aspirin, even without any history of asthma flares with aspirin use. Such studies suggest that, as a general rule, it is wise for asthma patients to avoid aspirin and products that contain aspirin, regardless of their past experience. Therefore, asthma patients should become familiar with common over-the-counter and prescription products that contain aspirin (see Table 2–3).

In addition, asthma patients who are sensitive to aspirin should also avoid a group of medications called the nonsteroidal anti-inflammatory medications, which are often used like aspirin to treat pain, headache, menstrual cramps, and arthritis. These medications can lead to reactions similar to those caused by aspirin in aspirin-sensitive individuals. It is for this reason that they are described as medications that can "cross-react" with aspirin. These medications include ibuprofen (Motrin, Advil, Nuprin), naproxen (Naprosyn, Anaprox), and piroxicam (Feldene). Table 2–4 provides a more complete list of the most common medications that can cross-react with aspirin.

Tartrazine (yellow food dye #5) can also precipitate asthma symptoms in some individuals, although this does not occur as frequently as with the other cross-reacting medications listed in Table 2–4. This food coloring is found in a number of soft drinks, cake mixes, candies, and some medications.

Some Products That Contain Aspirin

* Alka Seltzer

* Anacin Analgesic capsules and tablets (including Maximum Strength)—aspirin formula

* Ascriptin

* Bayer

* Bufferin

* Darvon with aspirin

* Easprin

* Ecotrin

* Empirin

* Excedrin—aspirin formula

* 4-way Cold Tablets

* Fiorinal

* Midol—aspirin formula

* Norgesic

* Percodan

* Sine-off tablets—aspirin formula

* Vanquish—aspirin formula

Table 2–3

Aspirin-sensitive asthma patients should avoid yellow food dye #5, as it sometimes can trigger symptoms that mimic the aspirin-induced asthma response. It is most important for all asthma patients to read labels carefully, especially in the supermarket.

Medications That Can Cross-React with Aspirin in Sensitive Individuals

1. All aspirin-containing products

2. Nonsteroidal anti-inflammatory agents such as:

   — Fenoprofen (Nalfon)   — Piroxicam (Feldene)

   — Ibuprofen (Motrin, Advil,   — Sulindac (Clinoril)
     Nuprin)

   — Meclofenamate (Meclo-   — Tolmetin (Tolectin)
     men)

   — Naproxen (Naprosyn,
     Anaprox)

3. Indomethacin (Indocin), phenylbutazone (Butazolidin)

4. Tartrazine (yellow food dye #5)

Table 2–4

Medications That Rarely Cross-React with Aspirin and Are Acceptable for Use by Asthma Patients

1. Acetaminophen (Tylenol)

2. Propoxyphene (Darvon)

3. Salsalate (Disalcid)

4. Sodium salicylate (Pabalate)

5. Choline magnesium trisalicylate (Trilisate)

Table 2–5

Acetaminophen (Tylenol) is considered to be an acceptable alternative to aspirin, since there are reports of but a few cases in which the use of acetaminophen has led to asthma symptoms. Table 2–5 presents some alternatives to aspirin that are considered acceptable for use by aspirin-sensitive asthma patients.

"Triad Asthma" Is When You Have:

1. Asthma

2. Nasal polyps (frequently associated with sinusitis)

3. Aspirin idiosyncracy (a drop in breathing function after taking aspirin or aspirin-containing products)

• People with asthma and nasal polyps should avoid aspirin, and
   products which contain aspirin or crossreact with aspirin.

Table 2–6

The most clear-cut association between aspirin and asthma symptoms is found in patients who have nasal polyps. This grouping of problems (nasal polyps, asthma, and aspirin sensitivity) has been termed "triad asthma" (see Table 2–6). These symptoms are frequently associated with sinusitis. There is no question that aspirin and aspirin-containing products, as well as products which cross-react with aspirin, should not be used by patients who have triad asthma. Chapter 17 discusses nasal polyps in greater detail.

For those individuals whose asthma is triggered primarily by aspirin, asthma symptoms usually begin at a later age, often arising for the first time after age thirty. As a group, these patients tend to be nonallergic, to need routine steroids more frequently, and to have a somewhat poorer prognosis for improvement.

The most practical management suggestion for all asthma patients is to avoid aspirin and aspirin-containing products as well as the nonsteroidal anti-inflammatory medications and tartrazine (yellow food dye #5). It is important to anticipate your medication needs if you develop a fever or achiness and to review with your doctor whether you should take aspirin. If you notice any change in your asthma symptoms with aspirin use, be sure to let your doctor know and avoid further use of aspirin.

QUESTIONS

1. One time I suddenly became short of breath and couldn't get any air. I passed out and didn't remember anything until I woke up at the hospital. I do recall having taken some aspirin for a headache. Could the aspirin have caused such a strong reaction?

Yes. If you're sensitive to aspirin, asthma symptoms that are triggered by aspirin can occur rapidly and be severe. It is very rare for an asthma patient to experience such a rapid progression to severe symptoms without being aspirin-sensitive. Knowing that you have had such a reaction, you should avoid not only aspirin but also aspirin-containing products and products that cross-react with aspirin, such as the non-steroidal anti-inflammatory medications typically used for bone and joint pain, fever, and headaches. One of these medications—ibuprofen (Motrin, Advil, Nuprin)—recently was made available over the counter. Avoidance of yellow food dye #5 is also advisable.

2. Should all asthma patients avoid products that contain aspirin?

There is no question that if you have nasal polyps along with your asthma, you should avoid products that contain aspirin or that cross-react with aspirin. It is still somewhat controversial whether aspirin should be avoided by all asthma patients regardless of their past experience with aspirin. Understanding the arguments for both sides, it seems wise that *ALL ASTHMA PATIENTS SHOULD AVOID ASPIRIN-CONTAINING PRODUCTS AND THE CROSS-REACTING MEDICATIONS*, since acetaminophen (Tylenol) is available as an alternative. The reasoning for this decision is that studies have found that some asthma patients with aspirin sensitivity are unaware of their problem. By avoiding this group of medications whenever possible, potential complications can be avoided. Sometimes it is necessary for an asthma patient to use one of these medications, such as for treatment of arthritis. If this is the case, then the decision must be reviewed with your asthma doctor so that any potential complications can be anticipated, possibly by being observed for several hours in the doctor's office or emergency room after the medication is taken.

SUMMARY: ASPIRIN AND TARTRAZINE (YELLOW FOOD DYE #5)

1. Aspirin and products that contain aspirin can trigger asthma attacks in certain individuals.

2. These attacks can begin suddenly and become severe within several minutes to several hours.

3. "Triad asthma" is the combination of nasal polyps, asthma, and aspirin sensitivity. A patient with triad asthma must avoid aspirin, aspirin-containing products, and medications that cross-react with aspirin.

4. Asthma patients who do not have triad asthma can also have asthma flares with aspirin. It is therefore advisable for all patients with asthma to avoid aspirin as well as products that contain aspirin and that cross-react with aspirin.

5. Aspirin-sensitive asthma patients should also avoid the nonsteroidal anti-inflammatory medications and tartrazine (yellow food dye #5)—see Table 2–4 (page 34).

6. Be a careful label reader and discuss all of your medications with your asthma doctor.

E. IRRITANTS

Irritants such as cigarette smoke, perfumes, strong odors, newsprint, and cold air can all trigger asthma symptoms in susceptible individuals. It is thought that these irritants cause asthma symptoms by stimulating irritant receptors found in the nose and in the back of the throat. These tiny nerve endings in turn stimulate the vagus nerve, which controls the tone of the airways. When the vagus nerve is stimulated by irritants, the muscles surrounding the airways then constrict, resulting in narrowing of the airways and asthma symptoms.

Most people with asthma are not allergic to cigarette smoke or other irritants. When you have asthma symptoms in response to these irritants, the allergic mechanism involving the mast cell does not come into play. Typically there is no IgE antibody against cigarette smoke and other irritants of this type. Rather than causing the release of histamine and other chemical mediators (as occurs in allergy), these irritants trigger the "twitchy" airways of the asthma patient to constrict, thereby increasing asthma symptoms.

Occupational environment can result in exposure to irritants as well as to allergens. It is important for you to consider whether your work place might be contributing to your asthma symptoms. Chapter 10 reviews occupational asthma, highlighting those occupations that clearly increase the risk of asthma symptoms.

While cold air is frequently a trigger of asthma symptoms, the impact on asthma of other aspects of the weather is not as clear-cut. Yet many patients report that their asthma symptoms tend to flare with an assortment of weather conditions, including rapid changes in temperature and barometric pressure, high humidity favoring mold growth, windy days favoring increased airborne pollen, and air stagnation favoring air pollution. Rain tends to reduce the amount of pollen in the air, although some mold spores are increased. It is important to recognize that certain weather conditions can serve as an irritant to your asthma, so that you can use good judgment in planning your daily activities.

As exposure to irritants is often unpredictable, it is best to have a management plan prepared in advance. The first step to take when your asthma symptoms flare from exposure to an irritant is to leave the area and remain as calm as you can. Inhaled asthma medications, available only by prescription, are fast-acting and are the best choice of medication in this situation. You should be sure to have the medication on hand in anticipation of needing it. Further suggestions for management in this situation are discussed in Chapter 5, which outlines a suggested management plan for asthma symptoms that begin suddenly, such as symptoms triggered by irritants.

QUESTIONS

1. Every time I go to a restaurant or a party where I am around cigarette smoke, I find that I start to wheeze. Is there anything I can do except avoid the situation?

Pretreating yourself with medication may be helpful. Using your asthma inhaler twenty minutes before you know you will be exposed to cigarette smoke may help you to avoid asthma symptoms. Other medications, when properly timed, can also offer relief. However, the ideal management is avoidance of the offending environmental situation.

2. Is there any test that can tell which irritants might cause my asthma to flare?

Unfortunately there is not. Your history of what happens in various situations is the only clue to defining which irritants trigger your asthma. You should discuss your observations with your doctor.

SUMMARY: IRRITANTS

1. Environmental irritants such as cigarette smoke, perfume, and cold air can trigger asthma symptoms in some individuals.

2. Irritants can cause receptors in the back of the throat to stimulate the vagus nerve, which can result in airway constriction and lead to asthma symptoms.

3. Asthma symptoms caused by irritants are not due to an allergy to the irritant. Rather, the irritant causes the already "twitchy" airways found in asthma patients to narrow, thereby causing asthma symptoms.

4. A plan of steps to take when irritants cause your asthma

to flare should be carefully worked out in advance with your doctor.

F. EMOTIONAL ASPECTS

Asthma is not a psychosomatic illness. The myth that asthma is "all in the head" has been a terrible burden for asthma patients to bear.

The tendency to develop asthma is often genetic. Although emotional upset can trigger asthma symptoms, it is clearly unfair for family members and acquaintances to view asthma itself as an indication that the asthma sufferer is in need of counseling.

However, if you find that your asthma is made worse by your emotional state, it is important for the doctor taking care of your asthma to know this. Often just talking things out with your doctor can help relieve any anxiety you might be feeling. If your doctor suggests that you see a psychiatrist or clinical psychologist, do not view this as an indication of failure. Your doctor and you must view yourself not as an asthmatic but as a person who has asthma. This is an important distinction because it encourages one to focus on the person, not just on the disorder. Possible approaches that can be taken include relaxation therapy such as biofeedback, family counseling, and psychotherapy.

Often patients report that they become upset by their asthma flares and that their asthma then becomes worse. These patients also report that they often try to ignore asthma symptoms and do not take medications, hoping that symptoms will disappear on their own. If this is the case with you, discuss it with your doctor, as this is a problem which should be addressed.

If emotional upset is one of the factors that triggers your asthma, it is even more important for you to understand your asthma and have a clear written asthma treatment plan prepared in advance by your doctor. This will give you confidence that you know exactly what to do if your asthma flares, which often helps to reduce your anxiety. Parents must be well informed about their child's asthma, so that they can help the child remain as calm as possible during an asthma flare.

Further discussion of psychological aspects of asthma is presented in Chapter 12.

QUESTIONS

1. I dislike taking medications for anything. I know when I should take my asthma medications but I often wait too long. You would think that I would learn, as I often wind up in the emergency room. Do you have any recommendations?

You should not mislead your doctor into thinking that your prescribed medications have been insufficient to control your asthma. If he thinks this is so, he might then have no alternative but to prescribe additional medications (possibly steroids) which may in fact be unnecessary. It is dangerous to develop a pattern of intentionally not taking routine medications, hoping that asthma symptoms will disappear on their own, since a prolonged delay in seeking treatment can potentially be life threatening. If you are frank with your doctor, he can propose a management plan to relieve asthma symptoms quickly so that you can avoid the emergency room. Discuss with your doctor your concerns about using the proposed medications, so that when the time comes to take the medications, you will use them.

2. My husband and I have disagreements often and we express our thoughts by yelling and screaming. We always make up but my daughter with asthma often starts to wheeze when this goes on. What should we do?

You should discuss this situation openly with your child's doctor, who may recommend family counseling. Professional counseling may help to reduce your child's asthma flares and also assist you and your husband.

3. My son is embarrassed to use his asthma inhaler at school, as he is afraid that the kids will make fun of him. What can we do?

First of all, explain to your son that asthma is nothing to be ashamed of. Then, ask your son's doctor to write a letter explaining that your son has asthma. In the letter he should outline the medications that may be necessary to control your child's asthma flares. It would also be helpful to attach a copy of your son's medication program. Be sure that specific indications or times for use of the inhaler are made clear. Copies of this letter should be given to your child's teachers (including the physical education teacher), coaches, and the school nurse. Once this is done, make an appointment to meet with your child's teachers to follow up on the doctor's letters. Often by clarifying any questions and opening a line of discussion, this will allow your child to use his inhaler at school as discreetly as possible so that problems with his classmates can be avoided.

SUMMARY: EMOTIONAL ASPECTS

1. Asthma is not a psychosomatic illness. The myth that asthma is "all in the head" has been a great burden for asthma patients.

2. Emotional upset can, however, make asthma symptoms worse. Therefore, be frank with your asthma doctor concerning the impact of stress and tension on your asthma.

3. If you tend to ignore asthma symptoms, "forgetting" to take medications and hoping that symptoms will disappear on their own, inform your doctor, as this can be a serious problem.

4. It is important that emotional aspects be considered in your asthma management plan. If psychiatric counseling is suggested, understand that your doctor is thinking of you as a person who has asthma and not just as an asthmatic.

5. It is important for you to have a clear-cut asthma medication plan available to you before asthma symptoms flare,

so that you will feel confident about knowing exactly what to do.

G. FOODS

There is no area of allergy so unresolved and tangled in confusion as food allergy. What is clear is that some foods (such as nuts and shellfish) can trigger immediate allergic responses such as hives, difficulty swallowing, gastrointestinal symptoms (including diarrhea, vomiting, and abdominal cramps), and breathing problems including asthma. The most serious consequence of food allergy is called anaphylaxis, a potentially life-threatening reaction in which there may be a drop in the blood pressure, swelling of the throat, a rise in the pulse rate, and the risk of irregular heartbeats and shock. Patients report dizziness and the sensation of passing out. If you have any of these symptoms after eating a particular food, it is essential that you report this to your doctor so that appropriate diagnostic tests can be performed.

Unfortunately, the only currently available treatment for food allergy is avoidance. If you have a food allergy, you should know in advance what to do if a reaction begins. All patients with a known food allergy should have antihistamines and Adrenalin for injection readily available, and should know how and when to use them. An Insect Ana-kit or EpiPen—Epinephrine Auto-Injector—are designed for emergency use of Adrenalin by the patient. Each requires a few minutes of instruction for proper use. Adrenalin is usually reserved for a severe reaction where the patient has difficulty breathing, difficulty swallowing, or the sensation of passing out. If you experience any of these symptoms or if you have given yourself an Adrenalin injection, proceed immediately to the nearest emergency room and then notify your doctor.

The mechanism for food allergy is the same as that for allergy to pollens. Namely, if you are allergic to a certain food, there is an antibody sitting on your mast cells that is specific to the food in question. When you eat (or sometimes just touch) that particular food, chemical mediators such as histamine are released from the mast cells, resulting in the symptoms described above. In order to be allergic to a given food, one must have developed the specific antibody for that food. This can be confirmed by allergy skin testing and by food challenges. Food challenges should only be performed by a physician skilled in this area, as there is always the possibility of a serious adverse reaction.

The accuracy of skin testing for foods has been questioned and is a matter of concern. Both positive and negative skin tests can at times be misleading. However, studies have shown that if a patient presents a clear-cut history of sensitivity to a food, a skin test (especially by prick technique) is often sufficient. The result can be confirmed by a double blind food challenge. In this test, neither the doctor nor the patient knows whether the food in question is actually given during the test, as the food is given in capsules or is in some way disguised. Because skin testing does seem to correlate with food challenges in the majority of patients who have a clear-cut allergic history to a particular food, the diagnosis can usually be confirmed with skin testing alone in this circumstance.

The RAST (radioallergosorbent test) profile is a blood test for allergies which provides results similar to skin tests. RAST can confirm food allergy in many instances. Although RAST is considered to be less accurate than skin testing, it offers the advantage of not exposing the individual to the potential allergen, since in rare cases this exposure can result in an allergic reaction.

The term food allergy is often used too loosely. There are adverse reactions to foods, called food intolerances, that do not involve the allergic mechanism. One such example is lactose intolerance, in which there is a deficiency of the enzyme necessary to digest milk. Patients with lactase deficiency experience bloating, abdominal pain, and diarrhea when they consume milk and certain other dairy products. This is clearly not due to allergy. Some other factors that have been wrongly attributed to food allergy include adverse reactions to food additives and preservatives, intolerances of foods such as wheat, and some psychological responses. Recently, adverse reactions to sulfiting agents, used as a preservative in many foods and medications, have been incriminated as an asthma trigger (see below).

Although obvious reactions to foods are relatively easy to confirm, the problem arises when trying to assess delayed reactions such as fatigue, achiness, irritability, tension, and a number of other vague symptoms that have been attributed to allergy. The mechanism of how these types of symptoms can be explained by allergy has never been clearly documented.

The leukocyte cytotoxicity test and similar methods that check for hidden food allergy appear to have questionable scientific merit. This particular test is considered by the American Academy of Allergy and Clinical Immunology to be a controversial technique. Despite these warnings, many patients continue to pursue their questions about food allergy through tests such as this. Some patients who are put on restricted diets as a result of information obtained from these tests do note some improvement. However, some of the diets these patients are placed on have been found to be nutritionally unsound. It is likely that the positive test results are often coincidental or the result of a placebo effect. However, it is clear that there is need for a greater understanding of food allergy. As soon as information of a more scientific nature becomes available, a better appraisal can be made of the array of symptoms that have been popularized as food allergies.

The information available today suggests that the chances are quite small that food allergies are a trigger for chronic asthma in adults. For children, elimination diets for milk products and occasionally for wheat products are sometimes successful. Certainly inform your doctor if you think that certain foods make your asthma worse. Even if diagnostic tests are negative, it may be wise to avoid the food in question as long as it is not nutritionally necessary. One group of foods that fits into this category is the mold-containing foods (see Table 2–7). If your asthma symptoms seem more pronounced after eating Chinese food containing monosodium glutamate (MSG), it may be wise to avoid it. Although there are no specific diagnostic tests (other than food challenges), foods containing sulfiting agents and yellow food dye #5 can sometimes be associated with asthma symptoms.

Mold Elimination Diet

Avoid the following:

- Beer and wine

- Baked goods that contain large amounts of yeast (such as soured breads, pumpernickel bread, and some coffee cakes)

- Buttermilk, sour cream

- Canned juices and canned tomatoes; other canned foods when not used immediately

- Cheeses of all kinds (including cottage cheese but not including processed cheeses)

- Cider

- Dried fruits (such as apricots, raisins, prunes, dates, and figs)

- Leftovers, especially fish or meat more than one day old

- Mushrooms

- Sauerkraut

- Smoked meats and fish (including hot dogs, sausages, corned beef, and other delicatessen items)

- Vinegar and foods that contain vinegar (such as ketchup, relishes, green olives, pickles, and mayonnaise)

Table 2-7

It is likely that in the near future more information will be available concerning the association of various foods with asthma. In the interim, follow the suggestions of your physician, avoid the temptation to explore gimmicky approaches, and recognize that, in view of the information available today, food allergy has been used as a catchall explanation for far too many problems. If you decide to explore unconventional techniques for treating a suspected food allergy, be certain that you remain in contact with your asthma doctor and that you stay well informed.

Sulfites

Sulfiting agents are used as preservatives in some foods as well as in some medications. They act as anti-oxidants, preventing the normal oxidation process which causes changes such as discoloration in fruits and vegetables. Sulfites keep vegetables and fruits looking fresh and crisp longer. Not uncommonly, restaurants apply sulfiting agents to lettuce to prevent it from looking limp and turning brown. Sulfites are often used on potatoes in restaurants to preserve their whiteness. Much of the controversy surrounding sulfiting agents stems from exposure of asthma patients to these agents, usually in a restaurant, resulting in a severe asthma flare.

Sulfiting agents are also placed on shrimp, often by fishermen while still on their boats, to prevent discoloration which makes the shrimp less desirable. Sulfites can also be found in most wine and beer as well as in some fruit drinks, dried fruits, baked goods, and processed foods. Most Americans unknowingly consume sulfites on a daily basis, especially in restaurants. Although harmless to most people, sulfites can present serious health risks for certain individuals.

Unfortunately, sulfites can also be found in medications, including bronchodilating solutions for nebulizers used in treating asthma. Efforts are being made to remove these agents. Currently metaproterenol (Alupent) is available as a sulfite-free solution only when used in the individual dosing (unit dosing) packages. Many of the other nebulizing solutions contain sulfites in varying amounts. In contrast, most bronchodilating inhalers are sulfite-free.

If you are sensitive to sulfites, you need to know that sulfites can also be found in cardiac medications, antibiotics, intravenous solutions, steroids (such as dexamethasone), painkillers, and some mood-altering medications. Some of these medications are not labeled to indicate that they contain sulfites, although efforts are being made to encourage proper labeling.

In addition to causing asthma symptoms, sulfiting agents

Some Products to Which Sulfites Are Commonly Added

- Lettuce and some raw vegetables served in restaurants or at salad bars

- Beers, wines, some fruit drinks

- Dried fruits

- Dips, especially those containing avocado

- Seafood (especially shrimp)

- Various processed and packaged foods (be a careful label reader)

- Asthma medications: Isuprel, Bronkosol, Alupent, and Metaprel multi-dose solutions for use in nebulizer (however, Alupent unit dose is sulfite-free)

Table 2–8

can rarely cause a severe, potentially life-threatening allergic reaction called anaphylaxis. Sulfites can also cause nausea, diarrhea, itchiness, hives, difficulty breathing and swallowing, as well as loss of consciousness. Several deaths have been attributed to sulfites. Reactions to sulfites usually occur within minutes of eating them, although delayed reactions of up to several hours have been reported. These reactions can also occur in individuals who do not have allergies or asthma.

Table 2–8 lists some common sources of sulfites. Careful reading of package labeling is important, since sulfites can be found in many foods and products in which you might not expect them. Sulfites are referred to in package labeling as sodium sulfite, sulfur dioxide, sodium and potassium bisulfite, and sodium and potassium metabisulfite. The Food and Drug Administration is reevaluating the safety of these agents. Although the use of sulfites by restaurants is still permitted, the Food and Drug Administration has requested that the National Restaurant Association ask its members to inform customers when sulfites are added to foods. Yet it is still important for you to inquire whether a restaurant uses sulfites if you think you may be sensitive to them.

QUESTIONS

1. Sometimes when I drink wine, I notice that I get a tickle in my throat and then start to cough and wheeze. Other times I am fine. Can you explain this?

Your report is not unusual. Doctors who treat asthma often hear of patients having problems with alcoholic beverages, including wines. Studies are under way asking the very question you raise. Issues to be addressed include whether the sulfiting agents used as a preservative in the wine are the culprit, or whether the mold content of the alcoholic beverage is causing asthma symptoms. The status of your asthma on any given day can also be a factor. For example, you may find the wine more troubling on a day when your asthma is more difficult to manage or on a day when the pollen count is elevated. The full answer to this question is not yet known.

2. It has become a habit for me to be a careful label reader, checking for tartrazine (yellow food dye #5). It surprises me how many products contain this food coloring. How important is it for me to avoid yellow food dye #5?

Patients whose asthma can be triggered by aspirin are more likely than others to have the same reaction from yellow food dye #5. It is clearly worthwhile for patients who have triad asthma (aspirin sensitivity, nasal polyps, and asthma) to avoid this food coloring. Yet recent reports suggest that the overall incidence of sensitivity to yellow food dye #5 in aspirin-sensitive patients is quite small. In general, asthma patients should be alerted to the potential association between yellow food dye #5 and asthma symptoms. Avoid products that contain this food coloring, especially for routine use.

3. I have noticed a marked reduction in my child's asthma symptoms since milk was removed from his diet. Should I worry that he is no longer drinking milk?

Since any restrictive diet can have nutritional implications, it is important that you work closely with a doctor experienced in making these decisions. In addition, your doctor needs to help you interpret the results of the diet. For example, some children have less mucus in their nose as a result of a reduction of milk in the diet. Therefore, the improvement you notice could be the result of less postnasal drip rather than a change in asthma symptoms. Clearly, there may be a need for calcium supplementation when milk products are avoided. If you have not discussed with your doctor the elimination of milk from your child's diet, mention to him the success of this restrictive diet and see what he recommends.

4. I'm frustrated about my son's asthma condition. He needs multiple medications to keep his asthma under control. I've heard about special food allergy tests that suggest either elimination diets or drops of allergic foods placed under the tongue. What do you think about these techniques?

Attempts at several medical centers to reproduce the claimed success of these controversial techniques in allergy have been unrewarding. You must understand this before proceeding in this direction. If you elect to seek an opinion from a physician who uses such techniques, be certain that you tell your asthma doctor and remain in close contact with him. Also be sure that you understand any risks associated with controversial techniques.

SUMMARY: FOODS AND SULFITES

1. Although certain foods and food additives can sometimes be associated with asthma symptoms, evidence available today indicates that the incidence of this is quite small.

2. Foods such as nuts and shellfish can result in an array of allergic responses ranging from itchiness, vomiting, and diarrhea to hives, difficulty swallowing, and difficulty breathing (including asthma symptoms). Anaphylaxis, the most serious reaction, can be life threatening.

3. The mechanism for food allergy is the same as that for pollen allergy as described on page 19. In order for there to be a true allergy to a food, there must be an IgE antibody specifically directed to the food in question. When the allergic mechanism is not involved, these adverse reactions are best termed food intolerances.

4. Skin testing is an imperfect but the best available means for diagnosing food allergy. If a patient has a clear-cut allergic history to a certain food, the diagnosis of allergy can usually be confirmed by a positive allergy skin test for that food.

5. Problems arise when trying to attribute to allergy a myriad of delayed reactions such as fatigue and irritability. Proposed methods for testing these delayed reactions (such as the leukocyte cytotoxicity test) have been classified as controversial techniques by the American Academy of Allergy and Immunology and have not been shown to have scientific merit to date.

6. With the information available to date, it seems likely that only in rare cases is food allergy a cause of chronic asthma symptoms in adults. However, if you suspect that you might be allergic to certain foods, you should mention this to your doctor. In addition, it has been reported that some asthma patients experience asthma symptoms as a result of sensitivity to sulfiting agents, yellow food dye #5, monosodium glutamate (MSG), and the mold-containing foods (especially wines, beers, and cheeses). Avoidance measures should be followed if you or your doctor suspects that you are sensitive to any of these agents.

7. Children are often placed on trial diets to see if elimination of certain foods (such as milk or wheat) reduces their asthma symptoms. It is important to emphasize that any dietary changes should be nutritionally sound. If necessary, supplements of missing nutrients should be given.

8. Clearly, more information is necessary to understand better the potential association between foods and asthma. In the interim, it is important to stay within the scope of sound scientific information and try to avoid the temptation of approaches that have been termed controversial by the American Board of Allergy and Immunology.

9. Sulfiting agents are used as preservatives in several foods and medications.

10. An array of symptoms, including asthma flares, can occur in certain individuals from sulfites. These reactions typically occur within minutes of eating sulfites.

11. Sulfites are used extensively on fruits and vegetables to keep them looking fresh and free of discoloration. Lettuce and potatoes are commonly sprayed with sulfiting agents. Large quantities of sulfites can be consumed with a restaurant meal.

12. Sulfites can also be found in processed foods, wines, seafood (particularly shrimp), and baked goods. Common sources of sulfites are summarized in Table 2–8.

13. Sulfites are also used as preservatives in various medications, including bronchodilating solutions for use in nebulizers. A careful review of your medications may be necessary if you are sensitive to sulfites.

14. Although this problem has received extensive publicity, it is not mandatory that restaurants inform customers that sulfiting agents are used. Thus, you should ask whether a particular restaurant uses sulfites if you think you may be sensitive to them.

15. Careful review of package labeling of processed foods can often identify if a sulfiting agent has been used. Sulfites can be listed under various names (see page 48).

PART TWO

✦✦✦✦✦

Asthma Management

◇ Introduction ◇

The basis for any asthma program consists of proper medications, along with suggestions for avoidance of factors that can trigger your asthma and, when appropriate, a program of allergy injections. The central issues involving medications concern which medications to use, when to use them, and how much to use. The proper use of the appropriate medications often reduces the need for stronger medications such as oral steroids, which when used long-term carry greater risk of side effects than other asthma medicines. Because asthma is a chronic illness and symptoms can occur at any time, it is vital that you understand the medications you so regularly use and upon which you so often depend. This background will assist you in better communicating with your doctor and understanding his advice.

The asthma medications can be summarized into four major groups (see Table 3–1):

- Theophylline—a derivative of caffeine and the most widely prescribed oral asthma medication in the United States.

- Adrenalin-like medications in both inhaled and oral forms—these are particularly appropriate for initial relief of an acute attack.

- Cromolyn sodium—a preventative inhaled medication for routine use or for use prior to exercise or prior to exposure to allergens.

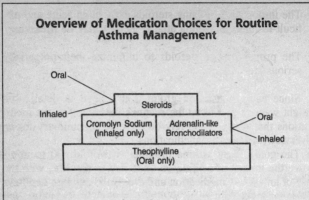

Overview of Medication Choices for Routine Asthma Management

Patients are often surprised to learn that there are only four major medication choices for routine asthma care. The medications are diagrammed above in pyramid form. Theophylline, cromolyn sodium, and the Adrenalin-like bronchodilators are all acceptable as first-line medication choices (depending on the patient's medical history). Theophylline appears at the bottom of the pyramid because it is the most widely used routine asthma medication. Steroids are the last medication that should be added for routine use.

Table 3–1

- Adrenal corticosteroids (steroids) in both inhaled and oral forms—oral steroids should be the last medication added to any long-term asthma regimen, since they carry the greatest potential risk of side effects.

This section will provide details on the effect and proper use of each medication and cover such topics as:

- The proper use of an inhaler and the risk of inhaler abuse.

- The advantages of inhaled versus oral medications.

- Determining the proper amount of theophylline to avoid side effects and achieve the greatest benefit.

- The importance of using steroids early in an acute and difficult-to-manage asthma attack, as they may be lifesaving.

- The proper use of steroids to minimize their potentially serious side effects.

Since each medication group is described in detail, you might want to read only the sections pertaining to the medications that you use and rely on the chapter summary for an overview of the other medications.

The goal of any asthma program is twofold: (a) to minimize the impact of asthma on one's day-to-day life, with the use of an asthma medication and avoidance regimen carefully designed by the physician with the patient's involvement; and (b) to avoid the need for steroids or to reduce the use of steroids to the minimal amount necessary, administered in the safest way possible.

◇ 3 ◇

Asthma Medications

A. ADRENALIN AND ADRENALIN-LIKE MEDICATIONS

Adrenalin. The first medication used in a hospital setting for an acute asthma flare is most often Adrenalin. The generic term for Adrenalin is epinephrine, and the two terms are often used interchangeably. Adrenalin helps to relieve acute asthma symptoms by opening the airways; this process is called bronchodilation. However, a negative effect of Adrenalin is that it stimulates the heart so that it beats faster. Adrenalin can also cause restlessness, paleness, headache, nausea, vomiting, and a sense of fear. Usually these side effects are transient. If you are given a shot of Adrenalin, you should expect to experience tremor and shakiness as your breathing improves—this is a normal reaction and should not cause you to be overly concerned.

Administration of Adrenalin. Adrenalin works quickly, offering relief within minutes. If the first dose brings only partial relief or if the wheezing increases again after the first dose wears off, the dose of Adrenalin is often repeated. This is typically done at twenty-minute intervals, with your doctor following your progress. Adrenalin injections should not be given more than two to three times in sequence, spaced by twenty minutes. Once the wheezing subsides, doctors sometimes elect to use a longer acting Adrenalin product called Susphrine to be certain that asthma symptoms are under control until other medications take effect.

Questions Raised by the Frequent Need for Adrenalin.

The frequent need for shots of Adrenalin raises questions about the asthma program you are following. Reasonable questions to ask include: (a) Did you wait too long before doing something about your asthma symptoms? (b) Did you know what to do when your asthma began to flare? (c) Do you have symptoms every day indicating that a routine daily asthma program would be appropriate? (d) Is your routine asthma program insufficient, suggesting that your present medications need adjustment or additional medications should be added to your program? (e) Did you break one of the rules about asthma? For example, did you abuse your inhaler by overuse, find that it no longer helped you, and then delay seeking treatment? (f) Did you follow your doctor's instructions exactly as directed or did you improvise? (g) Did you take an aspirin-containing product just before your asthma symptoms flared? Your answers to these questions should be reviewed with your doctor so that plans can be made to avoid or minimize the need for Adrenalin.

Adrenalin Dosage.

The usual dose of Adrenalin (1:1000 concentration) for adults is 0.2 to 0.3 milliliters, injected just under the skin (subcutaneously). For small children, the dose is determined by body weight. A reasonable guideline is 0.01 milliliter of Adrenalin multiplied by the child's weight in kilograms. As an example, if the child weighs 44 pounds, the Adrenalin dose would be 0.2 milliliters. This calculation is arrived at by dividing 44 pounds by 2.2, which is the number of kilograms per pound. Therefore 44 pounds equals 20 kilograms. Multiplying 20 kilograms by 0.01 milliliter equals the dose of 0.2 milliliters. The upper limit for Adrenalin for adults is typically 0.2 to 0.3 milliliters at a time. Needless to say, these calculations are given for the sake of completeness, as the dosing decision is made by the doctor. However, you now understand that you must know your weight or your child's weight so that the medication can be administered with greater speed and accuracy. Dosing adjustments are important to consider in adults who have heart, blood pressure, or thyroid problems, so be certain to emphasize these problems to the doctor.

Inhalation Treatments as an Alternative to Adrenalin. As an alternative in the emergency room to the use of Adrenalin, inhalation treatments using liquid forms of isoetharine (Bronkosol), terbutaline (Bricanyl or Brethine), or metaproterenol (Alupent or Metaprel) are acceptable and can be as effective as Adrenalin. These treatments are administered by a machine that aerosolizes the medication, called a nebulizer. Because the medication goes to the site of the problem (the airways) with less absorption into the body, side effects such as shakiness, nausea, and accelerated heart rate are much less. For this reason inhalation treatments are preferable to the use of Adrenalin for patients with heart, thyroid, or high blood pressure problems. In addition, children and needle-shy adults often appreciate avoiding an injection by using an inhalation treatment.

Use of the Nebulizer. An inhalation treatment is prepared by placing saline solution and the bronchodilating medication in the canister of the nebulizer. The patient then inhales the mist generated by the nebulizer for twenty minutes. Improvement of symptoms usually occurs within this time. The treatment can be repeated as often as every two hours in the emergency room setting. This same means of administering inhalation medication can be used at home with strict guidelines—the patient must not exceed one inhalation treatment every four to six hours without notifying his doctor. Home use of a nebulizer is appropriate for the difficult-to-manage patient who experiences unpredictable or severe asthma flares, who requires certain medications only effective by nebulization, or who otherwise requires frequent emergency room treatment.

Dosages of Nebulized Medications. The typical dosage for Bronkosol, one of the most common medications for nebulizer use, is 0.5 milliliters in 2–2.5 milliliters of saline. For Alupent or Metaprel, the dose is 0.3 milliliters in 2–2.5 milliliters of saline. Alupent is also available in unit dosing, with the saline and medication already mixed in a prepackaged container, which has the advantage of being sulfite-free (see Chapter 2). Terbutaline and albuterol are still not commercially available for nebulizer use.

ADRENALIN-LIKE MEDICATIONS FOR ROUTINE USE

Since Adrenalin can be administered only by injection and, ideally, under a doctor's observation, it is not practical for home or routine use. Over the years, Adrenalin-like medications have been developed which combine Adrenalin's key advantage of rapid opening of the airways with the practicality and convenience of oral and/or inhaled methods of administration. Doctors call this group of medications the beta adrenergic or sympathomimetic agents.

These medications, when used properly, are appropriate for routine use as well as for acute flares of asthma, often freeing the patient from frequent emergency hospital and doctor visits. These newer oral and inhaled asthma preparations, which include metaproterenol, terbutaline, and albuterol, offer the additional advantage of reducing the jitteriness and increased heart rate typically associated with Adrenalin. These newer agents are also longer acting, with a duration of action of up to six hours. It is the attempt to idealize these two key advantages—more direct action on the lungs with less effect on the heart, and a longer duration of action—that has triggered the development of new and safer asthma medications. Each of the Adrenalin-like medications will now be reviewed individually.

Ephedrine. When given orally, ephedrine is an effective but weak-acting bronchodilator (medication that opens the airways). In view of the newer medications currently available, however, ephedrine is considered to be an outdated medication. The disadvantages of ephedrine are increased heart rate and increased blood pressure as well as shakiness and sleeplessness.

Ephedrine is primarily used in a combination tablet which also contains theophylline and a sedative (such as phenobarbital) or a muscle relaxant (such as hydroxyzine) to minimize shakiness and restlessness. Examples of combination products containing ephedrine include Marax and Tedral. Although these products are still prescribed by many physicians and work well for some individuals, asthma specialists usually consider combination products to be outdated for several reasons: (a) They contain a fixed amount of theophylline, such that the dose of theophylline cannot be individualized. (b) In order to achieve the correct dose of theophylline, extra doses of the combination product must sometimes be taken, often resulting in side effects from excess ephedrine. (c) Sedatives are unnecessary for most individuals if the proper dosage of each of the medications is given. Moreover, sedatives should be avoided during asthma flares because they can suppress the urge to breathe at a time when breathing to the best of one's ability is crucial.

Products containing ephedrine are best avoided by patients with heart or thyroid problems. In general, there are a number of products available today that are superior to ephedrine and the ephedrine combination products.

Isoproterenol. Isoproterenol, formerly the most commonly used inhalation product, is an effective bronchodilator, acting within minutes. However, it stimulates both the rate at which the heart beats and the force of the heart's contractions and thus is an especially inappropriate choice for asthma patients with heart problems. In addition, isoproterenol's effect lasts only about two hours. It is for these reasons that isoproterenol has become a second-line drug for routine use.

In the emergency room, isoproterenol is still an acceptable alternative to Adrenalin when administered by inhalation. In severe asthma flares, unresponsive to all other conventional approaches, intravenous isoproterenol has been tried with reasonable success in pediatric patients. Isoproterenol is un-available in oral form because it is ineffective when taken by mouth. Isoproterenol is found in asthma inhalers such as Duo-Medihaler and Medihaler-Iso.

Isoetharine. Isoetharine is the generic equivalent of the products Bronkometer and Bronkosol, which are adminis-tered only by inhalation. Although isoetharine is not as strong a bronchodilator as isoproterenol, it has the advantage of hav-ing less effect on the heart and a slightly longer duration of action. Bronkosol is often used in the emergency room as an alternative to Adrenalin and at home by asthma patients who have sudden or frequent asthma flares.

Metaproterenol. Metaproterenol (Alupent or Metaprel) acts more directly on the lungs than isoproterenol and has a longer duration of action. However, it does not act as directly on the lungs (with less stimulation of the heart) as terbutaline or albuterol. In view of these distinctions, many asthma spe-cialists now favor albuterol or terbutaline over metaproter-enol, although metaproterenol is still an acceptable and effective choice.

Metaproterenol can be administered orally or by inhalation (via an inhaler or in liquid form used in a nebulizer). Its onset of action when taken orally is rapid, typically within thirty minutes, and its effect lasts up to five hours. It is well toler-ated by most asthma patients when taken orally, but it can cause shakiness, nausea, and rapid heartbeats in some pa-tients. Children like using the liquid form because of its pleasant taste. When used in inhaled form, metaproterenol acts within minutes and may last up to five hours. Along with Bronkosol, it has become one of the standard inhaled agents in the emergency room. Alupent brand unit dosing packages have the added advantage of not containing sulfites (see Chapter 2).

Terbutaline. Terbutaline acts more directly on the lungs and has less effect on the heart than metaproterenol. Terbu-taline works as rapidly as metaproterenol and is somewhat longer lasting. It is available in oral form and by injection (Bricanyl and Brethine), and by inhalation (Brethaire).

Terbutaline and albuterol (discussed below) both offer the advantage of acting more directly on the lungs (versus the heart) than the other Adrenalin-like medications. However, these medications can induce a greater incidence of shakiness, especially when the oral preparation is used. This shakiness is often of concern to patients using terbutaline and albuterol. Many patients are under the misconception that the shakiness (especially tremor of the hands) is caused by stimulation of the brain. This is not the case. The shakiness is in fact produced by stimulation of the skeletal muscles, and usually diminishes with time, reduction of the dose, or both. If shakiness is a problem for you, discuss this issue with your doctor. Some patients may have to discontinue using the medication, while for others the shakiness is a transient or tolerable problem.

Injected terbutaline is an alternative to Adrenalin in the emergency room. In theory, it offers the advantage of acting more directly on the lungs with less stimulation of the heart than Adrenalin. However, most physicians have concluded as a practical matter that injected terbutaline has little advantage over Adrenalin, except for the elderly or for patients with heart problems.

The newest asthma inhaler is Brethaire, a terbutaline inhaler which offers the promise of a quicker onset of action (within five minutes) with slightly less frequent side effects (such as tremor and nervousness) than does albuterol. However, this medication is still new and at this point seems quite comparable to albuterol.

Albuterol. Albuterol (Proventil or Ventolin), available for oral and inhaler use, produces rapid bronchodilation (opening of the airways) with little effect on the heart and a duration of action of four to six hours. It is the most commonly prescribed inhaler in the United States today. Albuterol is currently the standard among the Adrenalin-like medications against which new medications are compared.

In its oral form, albuterol has a rapid onset of action and duration of effect comparable to that of metaproterenol and terbutaline. As with those medications, albuterol in its oral form can lead to shakiness caused by stimulation of the skeletal muscles. This condition often passes with time or a reduction of the dose.

Indications for Use of the Oral Adrenalin-Like Medications.

These agents are useful as first-line or back-up medications, depending on the management philosophy of your doctor. The advantage of the oral agents is their rapid onset of action and the certainty that, when swallowed, the medication effectively enters the body (in contrast to asthma inhalers, which require proper technique for the medication to be effectively delivered). For persons with infrequent asthma episodes or for children for whom mastering proper inhaler technique would be difficult, these agents are excellent for bringing about rapid relief of symptoms without theophylline or before theophylline begins to work. Their usefulness is also evident for persons who have difficult-to-manage asthma requiring a back-up medication used routinely with theophylline.

Dosages and Side Effects of the Oral Agents.

Suggested dosages of the oral Adrenalin-like medications are listed in table 3–2. For these oral medications, use of the lower dosages reduces the risk of side effects. This is especially true for terbutaline and albuterol, since they seem to be associated with a greater incidence of shakiness. However, the shakiness caused by those medications is usually transient and passes if the medication is used for several days or if the dosage of the medication is reduced. Table 3–3 lists potential side effects of the Adrenalin-like medications in both inhaled and oral forms. Most patients report fewer side effects with the inhaled forms of these medications.

Asthma Inhalers.

Of late, great emphasis has been placed on administering asthma medications by inhalation because they then act at the site of the problem (the airways) and have less risk of the side effects often associated with oral administration. Such side effects typically include shakiness, rapid heart rate, vomiting, nausea, jitters, and headache. Table 3–4

Dosages of the Adrenalin-like Bronchodilators

Generic Name	Brand Name	Oral	Inhaled
Albuterol	Ventolin Proventil	Tablets: 2–4 mg, not to exceed 1 dose every 6–8 hours Syrup: 1–2 teaspoons (2 mg per teaspoon), not to exceed 1 dose every 6–8 hours	1–2 puffs,* not to exceed 2 puffs every 4–6 hours
Terbutaline	Bricanyl Brethine	Tablets: 2.5-5 mg, not to exceed 1 dose every 8 hours	
	Brethaire (inhaler only)		1–2 puffs,* not to exceed 2 puffs every 4–6 hours
Metaproterenol	Alupent Metaprel	Tablets: 10–20 mg, not to exceed 1 dose every 8 hours	1–2 puffs,* not to exceed 2 puffs every 4–6 hours
		Syrup: 1–2 teaspoons (10 mg per teaspoon), not to exceed 1 dose every 6–8 hours	Nebulizer solution: 0.3 cc in 2 cc. of saline
Isoetharine	Bronkometer (inhaler)		Inhaler: 1–2 puffs,* not to exceed 2 puffs every 4–6 hours

Table 3-2

Isoetharine	Bronkosol (inhalation solution)	Nebulizer solution: 0.25-0.50 cc in 2.5 cc of saline
Isoproterenol	Isuprel Medihaler Medihaler-Iso	Inhaler: 1-2 puffs,* not to exceed 2 puffs every 4-6 hours
		Nebulizer solution: 0.25-0.50 cc in 2.5 cc of saline
Bitolterol	Tornalate (new product)	2 puffs,* not to exceed 2 puffs every 4 hours; routine dose: 2-3 puffs* every 8 hours

*If 2 or more puffs are used, they should be spaced by 5 minutes.

Table 3-2 (continued)

describes the advantages of the inhaled over the oral Adrenalin-like medications.

Inhaler Abuse. It is most important to emphasize that asthma inhalers can be abused by overuse. An inhaler should be used no more frequently than two puffs up to every four to six hours (see Table 3-2). Your doctor should be notified if it is needed more frequently, as this may indicate that ad-

Potential Side Effects of
the Adrenalin-like Bronchodilators

- Nervousness

- Palpitations (increased heart rate)

- Shakiness (tremor)

- Headache

- Nausea

Do not overuse your inhaler or take extra oral medication.

Table 3–3

Advantages of Inhaled Medication
Over Oral Medication:

- Fast-acting—works within minutes

- Acts at site of problem (the airways), with less absorption into the rest of the body

- Less incidence of side effects such as shakiness and nausea

However, Inhaler Overuse Can Possibly Result In:

- Delay in seeking necessary treatment

- Irregular heartbeats

Table 3–4

ditional medications are needed. The major concern with inhaler overuse is that it may delay necessary additional therapy or emergency treatment. In addition, irregular heartbeats may occur with inhaler abuse.

Inhaler Technique. Proper inhaler technique is also essential. Figure 3–1 shows proper head and inhaler positioning

Proper Position of Head and Inhaler During Inhaler Use

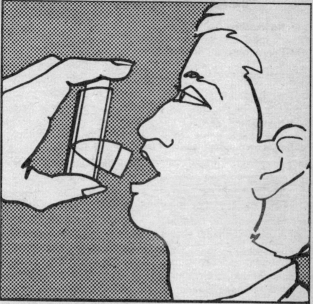

This illustrates the proper position of the head when using an inhaler. Note that the inhaler is held away from the mouth, not placed in the mouth. The mouth is held wide open. See page 68 for description of how to use the inhaler.

Figure 3-1

during inhaler use. The head is slightly tilted back to allow a straighter path for the inhaled medication. The inhaler itself is best held away from the mouth, not in the mouth as is often suggested. The reason for this is that by holding the inhaler away from the mouth, the medication is more likely to become aerosolized and pass into the air tubes, as opposed to hitting the back of the throat. However, it is also acceptable to hold the inhaler in the mouth, although this is a matter of debate. After exhaling as much air as possible, a big breath is taken in slowly while holding the inhaler a few inches from the mouth. Activate the inhaler just as you begin to breathe in. When you have inhaled as much air as you can, hold your breath a few seconds, preferably to the count of ten. Wait five minutes before using the inhaler a second time, which allows the first inhalation to open the airways for further penetration by the second breath of medication. Never activate the inhaler two times during one breathing maneuver. When your doctor instructs you to use two puffs of the inhaler, this means two separate breathing maneuvers spaced by five minutes.

Finally, keep the cover on your inhaler or carry it in a clean plastic bag when not in use. If you carry your inhaler uncovered in your pocket or purse, lint or dust can build up on the inhaler and possibly enter your airways during use. For patients troubled by arthritis who may have difficulty activating the inhaler, an inhaler attachment called VentEase is available.

Spacing Devices for Inhalers. If this technique is difficult to master or if you cannot avoid putting the inhaler in your mouth, ask your doctor about using a spacing device such as the cardboard insert used frequently for pulmonary function tests. This round cylinder is placed on the end of the inhaler and used as a mouthpiece, in order to provide the necessary distance from the back of your throat for the medication to become aerosolized. More sophisticated spacing devices and other special aids specifically designed for inhaler use are also available. They include InspirEase, Inhalaid, and Brethancer.

How to Tell if Your Asthma Inhaler Is Nearly Empty. Figure 3–2 demonstrates a simple method for determining how much medication there is in your asthma inhaler. This will assist you in determining whether it is time to ask your doctor to refill your prescription.

Over-the-Counter Inhaled Medications. Over-the-counter asthma inhalers such as Primatene and Bronkaid contain small doses of Adrenalin. Adrenalin is now rarely prescribed by doctors in the inhaled form, in light of the availability of the newer and improved inhaled products described above. In contrast to the newer inhaled agents, inhaled Adrenalin has the disadvantages of being short-acting

How to Determine if Your Asthma Inhaler Is Full or Nearly Empty

1. Remove the mouthpiece and place the inhaler in a container of water which is at room temperature.

2. An inhaler which is full will sink to the bottom. An empty inhaler will float on top of the water.

3. A partially filled inhaler will float somewhere in between. The higher the inhaler floats in the water, the more empty it is.

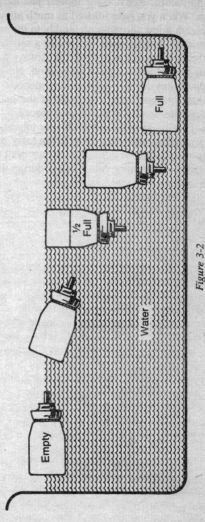

Figure 3-2

and of stimulating the heart rate and potentially the heart rhythm. As a result of their short duration of action, over-the-counter inhalers may be abused by too frequent use, despite the manufacturers' suggested guidelines.

The most serious drawback of over-the-counter inhalers is that for some patients they afford a small element of relief from asthma symptoms without necessarily fully resolving the symptoms. This minor improvement of symptoms often gives patients a false sense of confidence that their asthma is under control, thereby delaying a visit to their doctor for comprehensive care. *IT IS MY BELIEF THAT ALL ASTHMA SUFFERERS, EVEN THOSE WITH ASTHMA SYMPTOMS THAT TO DATE ARE INFREQUENT AND UNCOMPLICATED, SHOULD BE UNDER THE CARE OF A DOCTOR AND SHOULD BE PREPARED WITH A CAREFULLY DESIGNED ASTHMA TREATMENT PLAN.*

QUESTIONS

1. I frequently have to go to the emergency room for Adrenalin because my asthma gets out of control. Will it hurt me to have Adrenalin so often?

In all probability, no. In the emergency room your blood pressure, heart rate, and pulse can be monitored carefully, so the risk of side effects from Adrenalin is quite small. However, the emergency room doctor should be informed if you have any heart or thyroid problems so that he can consider the use of alternatives such as inhalation treatments or injected terbutaline, which in theory have less effect on the heart.

Your greatest risk in this situation is not the use of Adrenalin but the fact that your asthma is out of control. If your asthma attack is severe, there is a small risk that the attack could become life threatening. This is more likely to occur if your asthma symptoms are ignored and the symptoms are allowed to persist over a prolonged period. Without question, it is important to notify your doctor promptly if your asthma symptoms are not relieved by your routine medications.

Moreover, the emergency room is not the place for decisions to be made regarding your routine asthma care. You and your doctor should modify your asthma treatment plan so that, if possible, your day-to-day asthma symptoms can be better managed, thus averting the need for frequent emergency room visits. You must also be sure that you understand what to do as soon as your asthma flares.

2. Are there alternatives to Adrenalin shots so that I don't have to rush to the doctor's office or the emergency room?

Yes. Your doctor has exactly this goal in mind when he plans an asthma medication program for you. Alternatives to Adrenalin can include: (a) a bronchodilating inhaler which, when used properly, can offer relief within fifteen minutes, (b) an oral bronchodilator such as metaproterenol, terbutaline, or albuterol which can act rapidly within thirty to sixty minutes, and (c) an inhalation treatment with a home nebulizer using metaproterenol or isoetharine. The nebulizer is especially useful if attacks occur suddenly. The use of any of these medications should be under the instructions of your doctor. Additional medications, such as a product containing theophylline, should be available for use if the initial medication is not sufficient to bring your symptoms under control. Often the theophylline product is given for more sustained relief along with one of the first-line medications discussed above. When your asthma is unresponsive to the initial suggestions outlined by your doctor in your treatment plan, you should notify him so that alternative provisions can be undertaken early to avoid a severe asthma flare.

3. I have a history of rapid heartbeats even when I don't have asthma symptoms. Should I avoid taking Adrenalin?

If possible, yes. Adrenalin acts not just as a bronchodilator to open the airways but also as a stimulant to the heart's rate and strength of contraction. Since there are alternatives to its use, Adrenalin is best avoided in view of your medical history. The most simple solution is to try inhalation medications such as metaproterenol or isoetharine through use of a nebulizer. These products do not stimulate the heart as much as Adrenalin does. In addition, the inhaled medications offer the advantage of acting directly on the airways with less effect on the rest of the body. The newer inhalers such as albuterol or terbutaline have the least effect on the heart and could be tried as an alternative to an inhalation treatment. In the rare case where all forms of the Adrenalin-like medications produce irregular heartbeats, use of a rapidly acting product that contains theophylline should be considered. Without question, you might consult a cardiologist if you experience irregular heartbeats from using the Adrenalin-like medications. Your asthma doctor can then use this information to make the best possible choice of asthma medications for you. Consideration can also be given to preventative medications, such as cromolyn sodium or inhaled steroids, if indicated by your asthma history.

4. I use an inhaler which contains isoproterenol. Should I switch to one of the newer inhalers?

Yes. The advantage of the newer inhalers such as albuterol and terbutaline is that they act more directly on the lungs and have less effect on the heart, thereby reducing the small chance of producing irregular heartbeats. In addition, they have a longer duration of action, thereby reducing the chance that you will abuse the inhaler by overuse. At this time, inhalers that contain isoproterenol are no longer first-choice medications.

5. I hate the shaky feeling I get when I use medications such as terbutaline, albuterol, or metaproterenol, yet my breathing improves with their use. Are there any practical suggestions to lessen this adverse effect?

Yes. You need to understand that the jitteriness associated with these oral bronchodilators results from their stimulation of the muscles in the arm, as opposed to stimulation of the brain. The most simple solution is to substitute an inhaled bronchodilator for the oral bronchodilator you are now using. However, there is the reassurance that usually with time the jitteriness associated with the oral bronchodilator becomes less noticeable or subsides. Often the problem can be resolved by reducing the dose of the oral bronchodilator. If the oral bronchodilator is truly needed and there is no alternative short of steroids, then a muscle relaxant called hydroxyzine (Atarax or Vistaril) can be given. This combination is often successful. You might experience sleepiness when using hydroxyzine; therefore, be sure to exercise caution with activities that require full alertness. Often, a small dose of hydroxyzine (such as 10 to 20 milligrams) taken at bedtime is sufficient.

6. I prefer to put my inhaler directly into my mouth. Is that all right?

Although the directions that accompany inhalers still suggest that you place the inhaler in your mouth, it has become apparent that this technique causes much of the material to strike the back of the throat rather than to become aerosolized into the airways. You should learn how to use your inhaler properly (see Figure 3-1). As an alternative, a spacing device as simple as the cardboard mouthpiece used in spirometry or as sophisticated as some of the commercially available designs can be considered. Proper inhalation technique can make a significant difference in the effectiveness of the inhaler. You should not assume that your technique is correct unless it has been checked by your doctor.

7. When my asthma flares, I often have to use my inhaler every half hour. I know I'm not supposed to, but what else can I do?

If your asthma is out of control and you have to use your inhaler that frequently, call your doctor. Often in situations like the one you have described, your doctor will suggest that you go to the emergency room for an assessment of your breathing status, with consideration given to the use of alternative medications. Remember that the steroid medications take from four to six hours to work. Thus, when asthma is out of control, a quick-acting treatment is still necessary. This is usually provided with the use of Adrenalin or an inhalation treatment along with intravenous aminophylline.

In most cases, severe asthma symptoms do not begin rapidly. When your doctor carefully reviews your medical history with you, it usually becomes apparent that your asthma symptoms were becoming progressively worse and were neglected. Back-up medications may not have been used or may not have been available, and your doctor may have been contacted far too late to offer any suggestions short of the emergency room. These mistakes should be avoided in the future.

Inhalers are convenient to use and offer rapid relief. For

this reason they are frequently abused by overuse. Recent studies do indicate that the newer inhalers such as albuterol can be used much more frequently than the previously recommended limit, with little risk of side effects. However, since the most serious potential side effect of inhaler abuse is the risk of irregular heartbeats, which theoretically can lead to stoppage of the heart, it seems wise at this point to continue to limit use of even the newer inhalers to no more than two puffs every four to six hours. Fortunately, the likelihood of serious, potentially life-threatening side effects is small, but clearly inhaler abuse is frowned upon by all physicians.

The preferred inhalers are the newer ones such as albuterol or terbutaline, which are longer lasting and therefore less often abused by overuse, and which act more directly on the lungs with less effect on the heart, thereby reducing the risk of irregular heartbeats. Metaproterenol is also acceptable, although it does not act as directly on the airways as terbutaline or albuterol. You must know the limitations of inhaler use and abide by them. If you need to use your inhaler more frequently than recommended, your doctor should be notified promptly so that the need for emergency care hopefully can be averted.

SUMMARY: ADRENALINE AND ADRENALINE-LIKE MEDICATIONS

1. Adrenalin, which is the same as epinephrine, is usually the first medication used for asthma that is out of control, in both the doctor's office and the emergency room.

2. Adrenalin helps to open the airways rapidly. However, adrenalin may also cause the heart to beat faster, as well as cause shakiness, nausea, and vomiting. These side effects are usually transient.

3. Because Adrenalin's effect of opening the airways wears off quickly, it often must be given again at twenty-minute intervals, but should never be given in excess of three doses in succession. A longer-acting form of Adrenalin called Sus-

phrine is often used once wheezing has subsided, to prevent setbacks until other medications take effect.

4. An inhalation treatment using Bronkosol or Alupent is an alternative to Adrenalin. These treatments act rapidly and have the advantage of less side effects than Adrenalin.

5. While Adrenalin is used in asthma care strictly for emergency treatment, Adrenalin-like medications have been developed for use in nonemergency situations as well as for routine use. These medications include isoproterenol (Isuprel, Medihaler-Iso, or Duo-Medihaler), metaproterenol (Alupent or Metaprel), terbutaline (Brethaire, Brethine, or Bricanyl), and albuterol (Proventil and Ventolin). This group of medications combines Adrenalin's advantage of rapid opening of the airways, with the convenience of oral and/or inhaled methods of use. In addition, the newer products provide more direct action on the lungs with less effect on the heart, as well as longer duration of action.

6. Isoproterenol, once the most commonly used inhaled product, now is a second-line drug for routine use because it lasts only about two hours and has a greater effect on the heart than do the newer inhaled agents.

7. Metaproterenol, terbutaline, and albuterol offer the advantage of lasting up to six hours, with less effect on the heart than isoproterenol. In principle, terbutaline and albuterol both act more directly on the lungs (with less effect on the heart) than metaproterenol.

8. Asthma inhalers act directly on the airways, with less risk of the side effects often associated with oral asthma medications. Proper inhaler technique is important in order for inhaled medicines to provide the expected relief. Inhalers must be used no more frequently than two puffs every four to six hours, as more frequent use might delay necessary additional therapy or emergency treatment, or cause irregular heartbeats.

B. THEOPHYLLINE

Without question, the mainstay of most asthma medication programs in the United States is a theophylline product. Theophylline works by relaxing the muscles surrounding the air tubes, thereby opening the airways, and by preventing the mast cells from releasing chemical mediators such as histamine which lead to asthma symptoms in the allergic individual. Other effects of theophylline include an increase in the patient's heart rate as well as in the strength of the heart's contractions. Theophylline also causes stimulation of the nervous system and acts as a mild diuretic, causing an increase in urination.

Theophylline is found in many different products, and is available in both long-acting and short-acting forms. When used properly, most are fine products which bring about a similar result. Since theophylline is available in various strengths, the physician is able to adjust the theophylline dose to the appropriate amount for each patient. The choice of theophylline preparation is very important and should match the frequency of the patient's symptoms.

Long-Acting Theophylline. A long-acting theophylline product is appropriate for patients who have chronic asthma symptoms and require theophylline on a daily basis. The advantages of the long-acting products are the convenience of having to remember less often to take medication and of facilitating an uninterrupted eight- to twelve-hour night of sleep. In addition, when the dose of a long-acting product is properly adjusted, the amount of theophylline necessary to keep the airways open is more or less constantly maintained in the bloodstream. Some of the more common long-acting theophylline products are listed in Table 3–5. Some theophylline brand names include the designation "SR" (slow-release), "SA" (sustained-action), "LA" (long-acting), and "CRT" (controlled-release) which indicate that it is a long-acting form of theophylline. However, Theo-dur and Slo-bid, the two most commonly prescribed long-acting theophylline products, do not carry this designation.

Some Long-Acting Theophylline Products (Alphabetically)

Brand Name and Manufacturer	Theophylline Content in Milligrams
Choledyl SA (Parke-Davis)	256 and 384 mg tablets
Constant-T (Geigy)	200 and 300 mg tablets
Elixophyllin SR (Berlex)	125 and 250 mg capsules
La BID (Norwich Eaton)	250 mg tablets
Quibron-T/SR Dividose (Mead Johnson)	300 mg tablets
Respbid (Boehringer Ingelheim)	250 and 500 mg tablets
Slo-bid Gyrocaps (Rorer)	50, 100, 200 and 300 mg capsules
Slo-Phyllin Gyrocaps (Rorer)	60, 125, and 250 mg capsules
Somophyllin-CRT (Fisons)	50, 100, 200, 250, and 300 mg capsules
Sustaire (Roerig)	100 and 300 mg tablets
Theo-dur (Key)	100, 200, and 300 mg tablets
Theo-dur Sprinkle (Key)	50, 75, 125, and 200 mg capsules
Theolair—SR (Riker)	200, 250, 300, and 500 mg tablets
Theophyl—SR (McNeil)	125, 250 mg capsules
Theovent (Schering)	125, 250 mg capsules
24-Hour Preparations	
Theo-24 (Searle)	100, 200, and 300 mg capsules
Uniphyll (Purdue Frederick)	200 and 400 mg tablets (scored)

Table 3–5

Twenty-four-hour Theophylline Products.

The recent introduction of Theo-24 and Uniphyl offers patients the convenience of having to take theophylline only once a day. Although some patients can be successfully managed using a twenty-four-hour product, these products may not be appropriate for everyone. For patients who tend to metabolize theophylline rapidly, the medication may not last the full twenty-four-hour time period. Careful monitoring of your symptoms and your theophylline level is important if your doctor elects to use a twenty-four-hour theophylline product.

Long-Acting Products Should Not Be Broken, Crushed, Or Chewed. As the long-acting theophylline products are designed to release theophylline slowly over time, the capsule or pill should not be damaged or altered in any way. Some products are scored so that they can be broken in half. If a tablet does not have a marking that indicates that it can be broken, it would be a mistake to use a broken pill since all of the twelve-hour dose could then be released at once, resulting in side effects.

Short-Acting Theophylline. The short-acting theophylline products are appropriate for patients who have asthma episodes only occasionally, and who are free of asthma symptoms between episodes. When their asthma flares, these patients need a theophylline product that will work quickly (within one to two hours) to help relieve symptoms. These patients cannot wait until the long-acting products take effect. The major disadvantage of the short-acting products is that usually they must be taken every six hours. Some of the more commonly prescribed short-acting theophylline products include Slo-Phyllin tablets, Quibron, Elixophyllin capsules, Theolair tablets, and Somophyllin-T capsules (see Table 3–6). These products are also available in short-acting liquid form.

"Sprinkle" Theophylline Preparations. For years, young children who were unable to swallow pills or capsules could not take advantage of long-acting theophylline products, which were only available in pill or capsule form. With the availability of long-acting theophylline products that can be taken out of the capsule and sprinkled into food such as chocolate syrup or apple sauce, young children are now able to use long-acting theophylline. One of the advantages for children of the long-acting products is that the medication is taken only two to three times a day, versus four times a day for the short-acting products. This means the child need not be disturbed from an eight- to twelve-hour night of sleep to

Some Short-Acting Theophylline Products (Alphabetically)

Brand Name and Manufacturer	Theophylline Content of Liquid Form	Theophylline Content of Capsules or Tablets
Bronkodyl (Breon)	80 mg per teaspoon	Capsules: 100 mg, 200 mg
Elixicon (Berlex)	100 mg per tablespoon (nonalcohol base)	
Elixophyllin (Berlex)	80 mg per tablespoon (20% alcohol base)	Capsules: 125 mg, 250 mg
Quibron (Mead Johnson)	150 mg per tablespoon	Capsules: 150 mg, 350 mg
Slo-Phyllin (Rorer)	80 mg per tablespoon (nonalcohol base)	Tablets: 100 mg, 200 mg
Somophyllin (Fisons)	90 mg per teaspoon	Capsules: 100 mg, 200 mg, 250 mg
Theolair (Riker)	80 mg per tablespoon	Tablets: 125 mg, 250 mg
Theophyl (McNeil)	Approximately 225 mg per 2 tablespoons (alcohol base)	Chewable tablets: approximately 100 mg; tablets are scored so that they can be broken into fourths

Table 3–6

take medication. In addition to its convenience, long-acting theophylline maintains a more constant blood theophylline level, which makes asthma management somewhat easier. However, some children metabolize theophylline so quickly that they are not able to maintain a consistent blood theophylline level with a long-acting product. If this is the case with your child, a short-acting form of theophylline or more frequent dosing have to be used instead.

Advantages/Disadvantages of the Currently Available Theophylline Products

Long-acting products
Examples: Theo-dur, Slo-Phyllin Gyrocaps, Slo-bid

Advantages:
- Easier to remember to use because taken only twice a day (morning and evening)
- Allow 8 hours of sleep

Disadvantage:
- Do not provide immediate relief in acute situation

Short-acting products
Examples: Slo-Phyllin tablets, Elixophyllin, Quibron

Advantage:
- Provide immediate relief for patients who have infrequent asthma symptoms

Disadvantage:
- Must be taken every 6 hours around the clock

Table 3-7

Rectal Suppositories Containing Theophylline Are Not Recommended. Rectal administration of theophylline is not ideal, since the absorption of theophylline within the rectum is somewhat erratic and it is most important to know how much theophylline is actually in the blood. For this reason rectal suppositories containing theophylline are now rarely prescribed by asthma doctors.

The Reason For Performing Blood Theophylline Levels. Theophylline must be given in the proper amount. The reason for this concern is that there is no certain way of knowing how much theophylline an individual needs without checking a blood sample. Namely, if the same dose of a typical theophylline product is given to a group of people of the same age and weight, there is up to a sevenfold difference in the amount of theophylline in their blood at any given time because each person handles theophylline differently. One person's body may break down the medication rapidly while

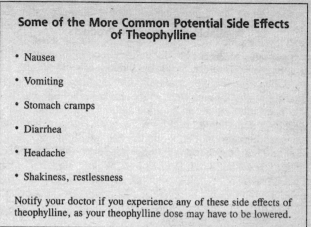

Some of the More Common Potential Side Effects of Theophylline

- Nausea

- Vomiting

- Stomach cramps

- Diarrhea

- Headache

- Shakiness, restlessness

Notify your doctor if you experience any of these side effects of theophylline, as your theophylline dose may have to be lowered.

Table 3–8

another person's body may metabolize it more slowly. Thus, the amount of theophylline that each person needs must be determined on an individual basis.

This is accomplished with the use of a simple blood test called a blood theophylline level. This test tells the doctor exactly how much theophylline is in the patient's blood at the time of the test. Doctors aim for a result in the "therapeutic range," which is the amount of medication which will provide most patients with the greatest benefit (in the case of theophylline, opening of the airways) with the least risk of side effects. The therapeutic range for theophylline is from 10 to 20 micrograms of theophylline per milliliter of blood serum.

Side Effects of Theophylline. As theophylline levels approach and exceed 20 micrograms per milliliter, the risk of theophylline side effects increases. Typical side effects indicating that your dosage of theophylline may be too high include nausea, diarrhea, vomiting, shakiness, headache, and increased heart rate (see Table 3-8). Some patients experience leg cramps from theophylline, especially at night. Lower potassium levels sometimes caused by use of theophylline or steroids can also contribute to this problem. If the theophylline level exceeds 20, there is a small risk of seizure, the most serious of the theophylline side effects. Fortunately this is a very rare occurrence. Theophylline levels of less than 10 are acceptable, as approximately 70 percent of the bronchodilating ability occurs with levels less than 10. However, if you need medications in addition to theophylline (especially steroids), you should be certain that your theophylline dose has been checked and is within the therapeutic range.

FOR THE DIFFICULT-TO-MANAGE ASTHMA PATIENT, THE THEOPHYLLINE LEVEL MUST BE WITHIN THE THERAPEUTIC RANGE TO BE CERTAIN THAT THE GREATEST POSSIBLE BENEFIT FROM THEOPHYLLINE IS ACHIEVED BEFORE CONCLUDING THAT ROUTINE ORAL STEROIDS ARE ESSENTIAL.

Some Patients Are Intolerant of Theophylline. Some people are unable to tolerate even low doses of theophylline, as theophylline causes them to experience unmanageable jitteriness, stomach upset, or headache. Some children become "hyped up" and are more likely to have behavioral problems when using theophylline, although most children are able to tolerate theophylline without significant problems. If you or your child cannot tolerate theophylline, discuss this problem with your doctor. If you do not have better results with the use of an alternate theophylline preparation, your asthma program may have to be modified to rely on medications other than theophylline.

The Importance of a Timed Theophylline Level. The time when the theophylline level is performed is also important (see Table 3–9). A theophylline level performed at the estimated time when the medication should be the greatest in the bloodstream is called the peak level. A trough level is the estimated time when the medication reaches its lowest concentration in the bloodstream.

A peak theophylline level should be taken if the doctor wants to know whether the amount of theophylline in the bloodstream is at a safe level, without risk of serious side

Theophylline Levels

- Peak Level—Checks whether there is too much theophylline in your bloodstream as well as whether the theophylline dose is sufficiently high

- Trough level—Checks whether there is rapid theophylline breakdown (resulting in asthma symptoms sooner than expected)

Table 3–9

effects; in addition, the doctor will also be able to determine if the dose of theophylline he prescribed is sufficient. Suggested times for determining the peak theophylline level are between the fourth and sixth hour for long-acting preparations such as Theo-dur, Slo-bid, and Somophyllin CRT, and between the fourth and fifth hour for Slo-Phyllin gyrocaps. Short-acting agents such as Elixophyllin or Slo-Phyllin tablets or liquid should be checked between the first and second hour after the dose is taken.

The trough level is of importance if one is having increased asthma symptoms earlier than expected at a time when the medication is wearing off. This can occur in some patients between the eighth to twelfth hour with Theo-dur, between the sixth to eighth hour with Slo-Phyllin gyrocaps, and between the fourth and sixth hour with the shorter-acting liquids and tablets.

With this background, it is easy to understand that careful evaluation of your progress with theophylline is necessary to be sure that you are getting the greatest benefit from this commonly prescribed medication. You should not assume, as some patients do, that you are taking the correct dosage of theophylline unless it has been checked with a timed theophylline level. If you experience daily asthma symptoms and need other asthma medications in addition to theophylline to keep your asthma in check (especially steroids), then a careful comparison of the pattern of your symptoms to your theophylline level is essential. Does your asthma act up between the eighth to twelfth hour after taking your long-acting theophylline? A trough theophylline level will indicate whether there is too little theophylline in your blood during this time period, and possibly point to the need for taking your theophylline closer together than the usual twelve-hour recommended dose. Do you still need steroids on a regular basis? If so, attention to detail in all aspects of your asthma medication plan is essential. Without question, a peak theophylline level in the therapeutic range (ideally around 15) is important in order to derive the greatest benefit from this medication. You need to know that your theophylline level is not above 20 to be sure that you are taking theophylline in a safe dosage range.

The Advantage of Products That Contain Only Theophylline. The older theophylline preparations such as Marax and Tedral have fallen out of favor because they are "combination" products (see Table 3–10). These products contain a fixed amount of theophylline along with an Adrenalin-like oral medication called ephedrine and a sedative such as hydroxyzine (Atarax or Vistaril) or phenobarbitol. These products do not allow the dose of theophylline to be adjusted independently. Since we now know that the theophylline requirement varies from person to person, it is clear that the amount of theophylline in these preparations may be too little or too great for an individual, depending on the person's body size and metabolism. Also, if one were to take an additional pill in order to increase the theophylline dose, one would also be taking additional doses of the sedative and the ephedrine. For this reason the current recommendation is to use products containing theophylline alone, so that your doctor can make appropriate adjustments to tailor the medication dose to your needs.

Check the theophylline product that you use to be sure that it is 100 percent theophylline. For example, some theophylline products contain guaifenesin, a medication which is thought to stimulate clearing of secretions. Whether guaifenesin actually does so is a matter of controversy. If the dose of a theophylline product that contains guaifenesin is increased, the greater amount of guaifenesin might contribute to nausea. A theophylline level is often helpful at this point

Some Combination Theophylline Products

Brand Name and Manufacturer	Ingredients of Liquid Form	Ingredients of Tablet Form
Marax (Roerig)	Per teaspoon (5% alcohol base): 32.50 mg theophylline 2.5 mg hydroxyzine 6.25 mg ephedrine	130 mg theophylline 25 mg ephedrine 10 mg hydroxyzine
Quibron Plus (Mead Johnson)	Per tablespoon: 150 mg theophylline 100 mg guaifenesin 25 mg ephedrine 20 mg butabarbital	150 mg theophylline 100 mg guaifenesin 25 mg ephedrine 20 mg butabarbital
Tedral (Parke-Davis)	Per teaspoon of elixir (15% alcohol base): 32.5 mg theophylline 6 mg ephedrine 2 mg phenobarbital Per teaspoon of suspension: 65 mg theophylline 12 mg ephedrine 4 mg phenobarbital	Short-acting tablet: 130 mg theophylline 24 mg ephedrine 8 mg phenobarbital Sustained action (SA) tablet: 180 mg theophylline 48 mg ephedrine 25 mg phenobarbital

Table 3–10

to determine whether the theophylline or the guaifenesin is the cause of the nausea. With this caveat in mind, guaifenesin itself does not contraindicate the use of these products.

Is Caffeine a Substitute for Theophylline? As theophylline and caffeine have chemical similarities, there has

been recent speculation regarding the effect on asthma symptoms of drinking several cups of coffee. Although one's theophylline level does not become greatly elevated by drinking coffee, reports have suggested that caffeine can be used by some patients as a substitute for theophylline if their normal medications are unavailable during an asthma flare. Despite these reports, it is wise to rely on medications specifically designed for your asthma.

Estimating a Starting Theophylline Dose. Initial dosing of theophylline does follow some general rules. For the short-acting theophylline products and for Slo-Phyllin gyrocaps, the routine initial dose is 3 to 5 milligrams per kilogram of ideal (not actual) body weight per dose. For example, a patient weighs 154 pounds and is within the range of his ideal body weight. To convert this to kilograms one divides 154 by 2.2, which equals 70 kilograms. Then multiply this by 3 to 5 milligrams per kilogram. The dosage range for a 70-kilogram person is 210 to 350 milligrams of theophylline per dose. The mathematical calculations are presented in chart form in Table 3–11.

The reason for reviewing this is to give you a general idea of the appropriate first steps in theophylline dosing. For the long-acting preparations such as Theo-dur, the initial dose for an adult should not exceed 6 milligrams per kilogram per 12-hour dose, although the actual starting dose is usually much lower. For example, a reasonable starting adult dose might be 200 milligrams every 12 hours. Unlike most adults, children are notorious in terms of their ability to break down theophylline rapidly. Therefore, initial dosing of theophylline for children is best determined by use of a theophylline level, as a child's requirement of a long-acting theophylline product can easily rise into the range of 8 to 9 milligrams per kilogram per dose. If your dose of theophylline seems high or low in comparison to these rules of thumb, discuss your theophylline dose with your doctor, as a theophylline level may be helpful.

Medications and Special Situations That Affect Your Theophylline Dose. Your theophylline dosage may have to be increased or decreased in accordance with certain situa-

Rule of Thumb Estimate of Theophylline Dose

Step 1:   Calculate your weight in kilograms:

$$\frac{\text{weight in pounds}}{2.2} = \text{weight in kilos}$$

Step 2:   Multiply by:

3–5 for shorter-acting theophylline products

6   for longer-acting theophylline products for adults; children need their dose checked by a theophylline level

6–8 for longer-acting theophylline products for children under age 12; however, children need their dose checked by a theophylline level

Result: An estimate of the theophylline dose to be used at the scheduled time

Caveat: Given the variability in theophylline metabolism from person to person, a blood theophylline level is still necessary

Table 3–11

tions, as specified in Table 3–12. The most common reason for altering your normal theophylline dose is the addition of erythromycin to your regimen. If this antibiotic is needed, your doctor may reduce your theophylline dose by approximately 20 percent. If you have any heart or liver problems, be sure that your doctor knows this, as your theophylline dose must be adjusted to compensate for these problems.

Some people find that they are more able to tolerate the irritation to the stomach often associated with theophylline if they take the theophylline product with food. However, some patients who require higher dosages of long-acting theophylline may develop higher theophylline levels when this medication is taken with food present in the stomach (especially food that is high in fat). Since it normally takes two hours for food to pass through the stomach, it may be important for you to avoid eating for two hours before taking high doses

Factors That Require Adjustment of the Theophylline Dose

Dose may need to be increased	Dose may need to be decreased
• Children • High protein diet • Cigarette smokers • Use of medications such as phenytoin (Dilantin)	• Older age group • High carbohydrate diet • Use of the antibiotics erythromycin or TaO • Other medications such as cimetidine (Tagamet), propranolol (Inderal), allopurinol (Zyloprim) • Medical problems such as liver failure, heart failure

Table 3–12

of long-acting theophylline. You should discuss this point with your doctor.

Use of Theophylline with Other Asthma Medications. Theophylline can be used at the same time as the Adrenalin-like bronchodilators. Often when these products are taken together, the combination of the theophylline along with an inhaled or oral Adrenalin-like medication is more effective than each medication taken alone.

Your Theophylline Dose and Choice of Product Must Be Determined by Your Doctor. You should *never* change your theophylline dose on your own. Above all else, never assume that because one theophylline pill helped, it is all right to double your dose or to take extra pills without your doctor's approval. This thinking can put you at great risk for developing theophylline side effects that could be serious. In addition, do not attempt to substitute a different theophylline product or a generic replacement for the brand of theophylline prescribed by your doctor without first getting your doctor's approval, as there are subtle but important differences among some theophylline products.

Theophylline has traditionally been the primary medication

Suggested Guidelines for Theophylline Therapy

1. Match your medical history with the appropriate preparation—e.g., long-acting agents if you have daily symptoms; shorter-acting agents if you have symptoms only occasionally.

2. Avoid combination preparations, as individual theophylline dosing is important.

3. Avoid rectally administered theophylline (erratic absorption).

4. Be sure your dosage is adjusted by your doctor to consider any underlying problems which may affect your theophylline dose.

5. A theophylline level (peak and/or trough) should be checked to assure proper dosing in difficult-to-manage patients and to avoid adverse reactions to theophylline.

Table 3–13

relied upon for asthma management in the United States. With the information now available to us, theophylline can be used even more effectively. Table 3–13 reviews the suggested guidelines for theophylline therapy presented in this chapter.

QUESTIONS

1. What time should I take my theophylline?

The simplest answer is that you should take it at the prescribed times. However, you should also understand why the timing of your theophylline can be important. For example, if you take a long-acting theophylline preparation and have difficulty with asthma symptoms in the middle of the night, it can be very helpful if you take your medication on a 10:00 A.M. and 10:00 P.M. schedule. The reasoning for this is that the theophylline will be on the rise in the early morning hours, which is around the time when you normally have problems. If you take a long-acting theophylline product at 10:00 P.M., the medication will reach its peak at approximately 4:00 A.M., six hours after it is taken.

A 10:00 A.M. and 10:00 P.M. schedule is also helpful for the patient who has trouble falling asleep with long-acting theophylline, as the theophylline is not yet at a meaningful level between 10:00 P.M. and 12:00 A.M., which are typical bedtimes. If someone were on an 8:00 A.M. and 8:00 P.M. schedule, the theophylline could well cause difficulty falling asleep, as the 8:00 P.M. medication could already be at a meaningful level by midnight.

Another point in favor of a 10:00 A.M. and 10:00 P.M. schedule is that the morning dose will peak at 4:00 P.M., the typical time for children to be engaged in their after-school athletic activities. By having the medication at its ideal level at this time, the risk of asthma flares will be reduced.

These examples emphasize the importance of the timing of long-acting theophylline products. Other dosing schedules may have particular advantages for you. These details should certainly be considered as they can make a great difference in how you feel on a day-to-day basis.

2. What is the best theophylline product?

There is no brand of theophylline that is the best, although some products are somewhat better than others at maintaining a constant level of theophylline. If used properly, each theophylline product can provide relief. You must try to determine your ideal dose of theophylline, especially if you need theophylline on a routine basis. Your asthma history also helps to determine the type of theophylline that is best for you. If you have asthma symptoms only occasionally, it would be better for you to use a rapidly acting preparation, as opposed to a long-acting one, which takes from four to six hours to work. On the other hand, a long-acting product is convenient to take and therefore the medication of choice for someone with routine asthma symptoms. Remember that combination theophylline products and theophylline given rectally should be avoided.

3. I've never had my theophylline level checked and I'm doing fine. Should I suggest to my doctor that my level should be tested?

Even though you are free of asthma symptoms and are experiencing no side effects from theophylline, it is a good idea to have your doctor perform a peak theophylline level to be certain that your theophylline dose is not excessive. Since everyone metabolizes theophylline differently, there is no way for your doctor to know that your theophylline dose is in a safe range without performing this test. If you are doing well with your current dose, there is no reason to increase it even if your theophylline level is somewhat low, as theophylline can be beneficial to some patients in levels below the usual therapeutic range. However, if you require medications in addition to theophylline in order to control your asthma, a careful check of your theophylline level is important to be certain that theophylline is being used as effectively as possible in your treatment. The proper use of theophylline may make it possible to reduce or eliminate the need for other medications, especially steroids. In this setting, it is essential to check your theophylline level in order to determine the dose which is sufficient to bring the theophylline level within the therapeutic range (a theophylline level of 10 to 20).

If you are experiencing any of the theophylline side effects such as headache, nausea, or diarrhea, a peak theophylline level should be performed. A peak theophylline level checks the amount of theophylline at the estimated time when the greatest amount of medication is in the bloodstream. Since long-acting and short-acting theophylline products reach their peak at different times, the timing of when the theophylline level is performed is important.

4. I've tried all the theophylline preparations and they all make me sick. What should I do?

This can be a troublesome problem. Some patients are unable to take advantage of theophylline because of intolerance of side effects, even at lower dosage ranges. Work with your doctor to find a dosing schedule using lower theophylline dosages taken more frequently. Some patients have good results using a theophylline product such as Choledyl, which is thought to be better tolerated by the gastrointestinal tract (see Table 3–14). If these measures prove unrewarding, you will probably have to switch to a medication program that does

An Alternative to Theophylline

Brand Name and Manufacturer	Ingredients of Liquid Form	Ingredients of Tablet Form
Choledyl (Parke-Davis)	Per teaspoon of elixir (20% alcohol base):	Short-acting tablets:
• Advantage—better tolerated by the gastrointestinal tract than theophylline by some individuals	100 mg oxitriphylline (approximately equivalent to 64 mg theophylline)	100 mg or 200 mg oxitriphylline (approximately equivalent to 64 mg or 128 mg theophylline, respectively)
	Per teaspoon of pediatric syrup:	Sustained action (SA) tablets:
	50 mg oxitriphylline (approximately equivalent to 32 mg theophylline)	400 mg or 600 mg oxitriphylline (approximately equivalent to 256 mg or 384 mg theophylline, respectively)

Table 3-14

not use theophylline. If, on the other hand, your problem with theophylline involves shakiness, oftentimes the discomfort can be resolved by the use of a mild relaxant such as hydroxyzine (Atarax or Vistaril). However, during an asthma attack you should avoid using hydroxyzine and other medications such as sleeping pills that can be sedating. *NEVER TAKE A SEDATIVE TO HELP YOU SLEEP IF YOU ARE NOT BREATHING WELL, AS THE SEDATIVE MAY MAKE YOU TOO SLEEPY AND SUPPRESS YOUR DRIVE TO BREATHE. ONLY THE UNINFORMED PATIENT ASKS FOR A SLEEPING PILL WHEN HIS ASTHMA FLARES. THE RESULT CAN BE FATAL.*

5. When my asthma gets worse, I just double my dose of theophylline. Is that all right to do?

No. Any changes that you make with regard to your medications must be under your doctor's supervision. By doubling your theophylline dose on your own, it is likely that you have increased the chance of developing theophylline side effects, the most serious of which is seizure. Details of exactly what to do if your asthma symptoms flare should be worked out beforehand and written down to avoid any errors or misunderstandings.

6. My child is taking theophylline routinely and his asthma is no better. What should I do?

Even though your child may be taking an appropriate theophylline medication, the dosage may not be appropriate. It is very common for children to be rapid metabolizers of theophylline. Therefore, your child may require large doses to derive any benefit. The simplest way to resolve this problem is to ask your child's doctor to determine your child's peak theophylline level, to see if there is sufficient theophylline in the bloodstream to be effective.

SUMMARY: THEOPHYLLINE

1. Theophylline relaxes the muscles surrounding the air tubes, thereby helping to relieve asthma symptoms.

2. Theophylline products can be either long-acting or short-acting. Each has a particular usefulness. The long-acting products offer convenience and an eight- to twelve-hour interval between doses for an uninterrupted night of sleep. The short-acting products act more rapidly, and are more appropriate for individuals who have asthma symptoms only rarely and need rapid relief (because they are not using any routine asthma medications). Theophylline products lasting twenty-four hours are also available and are appropriate for some people.

3. Since there is no standard dose of theophylline that is correct for everyone, the proper dose must be determined on an individual basis. This is done through the use of a simple blood test called a theophylline level. This test

should be performed if (a) you are having side effects from theophylline, (b) your theophylline is not lasting long enough, or (c) you require multiple medications (especially steroids) to control your symptoms. The appropriate time of day for performing a theophylline level depends upon which theophylline preparation you are using and what information your doctor is looking for.

4. Side effects of theophylline include nausea, headache, diarrhea, and jitteriness. If you have any of these symptoms, you should notify your doctor as soon as possible, as your dosage of theophylline may need to be adjusted downward. Note the time you took your theophylline and the time you first noticed symptoms. Your doctor may want to check your peak theophylline level. Never increase your theophylline dose without first consulting with your doctor.

C. CROMOLYN SODIUM (INTAL)

Cromolyn sodium is a derivative of an eastern Mediterranean plant. Although how it works is not exactly clear, cromolyn sodium is an effective asthma medication for some individuals. One theory is that it stabilizes the mast cell, preventing mast cell products (mediators) such as histamine from triggering asthma. Since the mechanism for allergic asthma involves the mast cell, cromolyn has been thought of as an effective product primarily for those individuals whose asthma is precipitated by allergy. However, this limitation has been shown to be inaccurate, as cromolyn can be an effective preventative medication that reduces the reactivity ("twitchiness") of the airways regardless of precipitating factor. Above all, cromolyn is a nonsteroid agent and is usually not associated with significant side effects. For this reason it is a reasonable choice for many asthma patients.

Indications for Its Use. Cromolyn is useful as a pretreatment medication for asthma triggered by exercise, cold air, and allergens to which you know you will be exposed, such as animal dander. Cromolyn can also be considered as an alternative for individuals who are intolerant of the side effects of theophylline and the Adrenalin-like bronchodilators.

Without question, cromolyn deserves serious consideration in any asthma program, especially if the alternative is oral steroids. Cromolyn may well be the best medication choice for many individuals, serving as the mainstay of their routine asthma programs instead of theophylline. It is a misconception that cromolyn is effective only in children.

Cromolyn Is an Inhaled Medication. Until recently, cromolyn was most commonly prescribed as a dry powder in capsule form and inhaled into the lungs using a spinhaler, an inhaler specifically designed for cromolyn use. Cromolyn is not well absorbed by the stomach, and the capsules are not designed to be swallowed. A cromolyn inhaler has recently become available and is in widespread use. The technique for its use is the same as for the bronchodilating inhalers (see page 18). Cromolyn is also available as a solution which can be used in a nebulizer, a machine which creates a mist which is easily inhaled. This means of administration is especially appropriate for children too young to master proper inhaler technique.

Lactose in the cromolyn powder can irritate the throat. Although some of the cromolyn powder is inadvertently swallowed during inhalation, the amount is usually so small that it causes little or no problem for the lactose-intolerant individual.

Spinhaler Technique. Place the cromolyn capsule in the spinhaler with the yellow side down. Reassemble the spinhaler, and pass the gray movable sleeve down toward the mouthpiece and then up one time only, so that the capsule within the spinhaler is pierced and ready for inhalation. The same inhalation technique used for a bronchodilating inhaler is used for the spinhaler, except that with the spinhaler, the mouthpiece is placed directly in your mouth (see page 68 on inhaler technique). With the spinhaler held away from your mouth, breathe out slowly, emptying your lungs of air. Then place the spinhaler mouthpiece directly in your mouth with your head held back and take in as big a breath as possible.

It is your breath that activates the spinhaler. It is the timing and depth of your breath that carries the cromolyn to your lungs most effectively. You will hear a rotary sound when you activate the spinhaler properly. Hold your breath for a few seconds after inhaling the powder, to allow contact of the powder with your airways. When you exhale, don't breathe out into the inhaler. Although most of the cromolyn will be breathed in with the first inhalation, several inhalations may be necessary to empty completely one capsule.

Whistle Attachment. A whistle can be attached to the spinhaler to help confirm proper technique. It is especially useful for children. Children who are first learning about spinhalers tend to blow air directly into the spinhaler. As mentioned, cromolyn powder is taken in via the spinhaler only when the patient inhales. The whistle works only when you inhale, not when you blow out into the spinhaler. In addition, the whistle blows louder when you take in a fuller breath. Often children learn to master spinhaler technique more rapidly when this attachment is added.

Cromolyn Liquid for Nebulization. The availability of cromolyn in liquid form has added this useful medication as a potential choice for children who are too young or unable to master proper spinhaler technique. The material comes in a slender glass tube which, when opened, is placed directly into the nebulizer bulb. The mist created when the nebulizer is turned on is breathed in until the material is completely inhaled.

Dosage. For the new cromolyn inhaler the dosage is two puffs spaced four times throughout the day. The typical dose of cromolyn administered via a spinhaler is one capsule (20 milligrams) inhaled four times a day, for a total of 80 milligrams. This dose can be reduced once a satisfactory response to cromolyn has been achieved. Often it is possible for children to take cromolyn only three times a day—in the early morning, after school, and at bedtime, thus avoiding the use of cromolyn at school. As mentioned, cromolyn is often taken after using a bronchodilating inhaler such as albuterol to allow the cromolyn a clear passageway into the lungs.

For liquid cromolyn solution used in the nebulizer, the typical dose is two to four inhalation treatments a day. Cromolyn can also be used after an inhalation treatment of a bronchodilating medication such as metaproterenol or isoetharine, under the same principle of first opening the airways to allow the best possible access for the cromolyn. The major drawback of liquid cromolyn is the impracticality of using the nebulizing equipment when you are not at home.

If used as a preexercise preventative treatment, cromolyn is best taken fifteen to twenty minutes before exercise, and its effect should last for at least three hours. However, if you forget to pretreat yourself in advance, you can still use cromolyn just prior to exercise. Cromolyn will not block exercise-induced asthma once wheezing begins.

Cromolyn can also be used to prevent asthma caused by a foreseeable exposure to an allergen, such as a visit at the home of a friend who has a pet. In this setting cromolyn is best taken thirty minutes before exposure. If cromolyn is taken to prevent asthma during a spring or fall pollen season, it should be initiated at least one week before the start of the pollen season.

Special Instructions. It is preferable if cromolyn is introduced when you are feeling well, with no asthma symptoms. If your asthma is not under control, cromolyn can irritate your airways and cause your asthma to flare. If cromolyn is first used in this setting, you may incorrectly conclude that cromolyn is not a good medication choice for you.

Most doctors suggest using a bronchodilating inhaler just prior to using cromolyn, to allow cromolyn better access to the airways. This combination of medications offers the advantage of acting at the site of the problem (the airways), without causing significant side effects such as shakiness or nausea often associated with oral medications. The combination of cromolyn preceded by a bronchodilating inhaler is worthy of a trial in a child who gets "hyped up" with theophylline or other oral asthma medications. The decision as to the use of cromolyn in your case should be discussed with your doctor.

If you now use cromolyn only prior to exercise, ask your doctor if you could use it in other circumstances when your asthma typically flares—for example, before exposure to cold air or to pets. Its routine use by allergic individuals who are not diligent in environmental precautions may also prove worthwhile.

When cromolyn is introduced on a trial basis it should be used routinely for six weeks, as this amount of time is necessary to assess its full benefit. Therefore, do not be discouraged and discontinue its use if you find that cromolyn does not bring about dramatic improvement right away.

When taking cromolyn, you need to know what to do if your asthma flares. Cromolyn is a preventative medication, not a medication to which you should turn when your asthma flares. A back-up program is essential. A medication that contains theophylline (if you are not already using one) or an inhaled or oral Adrenalin-like bronchodilator is an appropriate first step. The exact sequence of what you should do is essential; these steps should be worked out in advance with your doctor. As you will see in later sections of this book, the back-up program should be written down to avoid confusion, as there may be a lapse of time until it is actually needed. Above all, if your back-up program does not provide relief, you must promptly notify your doctor.

Side Effects. Cromolyn is essentially free of side effects in most individuals. To date, there are no clear-cut long-term side effects associated with its routine use. The most commonly reported side effect is irritation of the throat caused by the powder. This is often overcome by rinsing the mouth with warm water after using the spinhaler. Some asthma patients notice that their asthma is triggered by the irritating effect of the powder. Proper spinhaler technique and the use of a bronchodilating inhaler before using the spinhaler often resolve this problem.

Other adverse reactions that have been reported from the use of cromolyn include hives, swelling, nausea, diarrhea, headache, and behavioral changes as well as seizure and dizziness. These reactions are quite rare and may all have been coincidental. As cromolyn is extremely well tolerated by most asthma patients, concern for side effects that are so unusual should not preclude this medication from consideration. At this time, the potential benefit from its use clearly outweighs any of the reported risks, especially in view of their low probability.

Cromolyn During Pregnancy. Cromolyn is best avoided during pregnancy. It has been used in Europe during pregnancy by a limited number of women with no reported birth defects. However, since it has not been used extensively by pregnant women and since there are alternatives during pregnancy (theophylline in particular), cromolyn should be avoided during pregnancy.

QUESTIONS

1. Whenever I use cromolyn I start to wheeze. Should I stop the medication?

No. You should first report this observation to your doctor. In all likelihood, your doctor will review your spinhaler technique to be sure that you are using the inhaler correctly. A frequent mistake in inhaler use is that the patient's head is not tilted backward, thus failing to provide a straight pathway for the medication to follow. With the head in the normal upright position, the inhaled medication is more likely to strike the back of the throat and, by its irritant action, trigger asthma symptoms. This mechanism involves irritant receptors located in the back of the throat which, when stimulated by an irritant, can trigger the vagus nerve (which normally controls the size of the airways) to constrict the airways.

Your doctor may also consider the use of a bronchodilating inhaler prior to using cromolyn to open the airways and allow the cromolyn better access to the airways. Your doctor will also assess your overall asthma condition to determine if your asthma is under sufficient control to allow cromolyn the chance to work. On occasion, another asthma medication may be added for a short time period to improve your breathing status and thus allow your doctor to assess more fairly your response to cromolyn.

2. My son simply cannot master the spinhaler technique. What are the alternatives?

The new cromolyn inhaler is probably the easiest solution for your son. Be sure that he uses proper inhaler technique (see page 68). If he wants to try to continue using his spinhaler, the addition of a whistle attachment makes the use of the spinhaler more fun and also will give him positive feedback when his spinhaler technique is correct. As he takes a big breath in while using the spinhaler, the whistle sounds. If he blows into the spinhaler as he would typically do with a whistle, the whistle makes no sound. Another alternative is liquid cromolyn used in a nebulizer. The only disadvantage of its use is the inconvenience of being limited to home use because of the need for the nebulizer equipment.

3. I understand that cromolyn is best used four times a day. However, I do not have routine daily asthma symptoms. I notice my asthma only when I exercise or when I'm around my sister's cat. Is cromolyn a reasonable choice for me?

Your question should be reviewed with your doctor to determine whether your breathing status usually is within normal range. Your doctor will examine your chest and give you a breathing test called spirometry, which determines if airway obstruction exists on a routine basis. If these studies indicate that your breathing is normally satisfactory, the focus should then be on preexposure and preexercise treatment regimens. Cromolyn is one of several choices of medications that can be used in this manner without using the medication routinely. For cromolyn to work it must be taken before the exercise or exposure occurs. If it is used after wheezing has begun, it will offer no protective benefit. Once your asthma has started to flare, your doctor probably will suggest a bronchodilating inhaler such as metaproterenol, terbutaline, or albuterol. These inhalers can also be used instead of cromolyn in pretreatment situations. Clearly, it is important to review your pretreatment plan with your doctor so that you can derive the greatest benefit from each of your medications.

4. When I start to wheeze, I find that using cromolyn is of little benefit. Why is that?

Cromolyn is a preventative medication which works best when taken for an extended period of time. It does not work like the bronchodilating inhalers, which afford an immediate sense of relief by opening the airways. Cromolyn instead reduces the "twitchiness" of the airways so that the airways react less to irritants and allergens. You must have the correct expectations for each of your medications. Cromolyn is not the medication to turn to during an asthma flare. Finally, it is important for you to have a carefully prepared medication plan to use when your asthma flares. This avoids guessing on your own what to do.

5. If I'm doing well using a theophylline product and a bronchodilating inhaler, should I ask my doctor if I should switch to cromolyn?

No. The goals of any asthma program are to avoid the frequent need for emergency doctor and hospital visits, to avoid the frequent need for steroids, and to allow you to go about your activities with as little inconvenience as possible. If these goals are being met and you are free from side effects with your present medication program, there is no need to change your program or to consider alternative medications such as cromolyn.

6. To control my asthma so that I can go about my routine activities, my asthma medication program includes a theophylline product, a bronchodilating inhaler, and steroids taken every other day. Is cromolyn the right medication for me?

It is impossible to predict with certainty who will have good results with cromolyn. Without question, your routine need for steroids is a matter of concern, although the risk of steroid side effects is far less with steroids used every other day rather than every day. A close working relationship with your doctor is essential. You should be certain that you are getting the greatest possible benefit from each of your non-steroid medications. For example, your theophylline level should be in the therapeutic range (10 to 20), and you should be using proper inhaler technique. If your nonsteroid medications are being properly used and the need for steroids persists, the use of other nonsteroid medications such as cromolyn can be considered, in the hope of reducing or possibly discontinuing the use of oral steroids.

SUMMARY: CROMOLYN SODIUM (INTAL)

1. Cromolyn sodium is an effective preventative medication for some asthma patients and deserves serious consideration in any asthma program, especially if the alternative is the use of steroids.

2. Cromolyn is an effective pretreatment (preventative) medication choice for (a) exercise-induced asthma, (b) cold air-induced asthma, and (c) asthma triggered by a foreseeable exposure to an allergen such as cigarette smoke or animals. It is an alternative medication for those individuals who cannot tolerate the side effects of theophylline or the Adrenalin-like medications.

3. Cromolyn is an inhaled (not an oral) product. Recently it has become available in inhaler form. It is also available as a powder used with an inhaler called a spinhaler or as a nebulizing liquid ideal for pediatric use.

4. Proper spinhaler technique is critical to the successful use of cromolyn. Often a bronchodilating inhaler is used before cromolyn to open the airways, thus allowing better access for the cromolyn.

5. Cromolyn should be first introduced when you are feeling well, for a six-week trial period. It is important to know what medications to turn to if your asthma flares while using cromolyn, since cromolyn is a *preventative* medication that is not designed to control acute asthma symptoms.

6. Cromolyn is essentially free of side effects, although it can irritate the airways and trigger a cough or, in rare

cases, asthma flares. However, it is not recommended for use during pregnancy because of insufficient testing.

D. STEROIDS

Without question, the topic of steroids sparks the greatest concern among asthma patients. And this is rightfully so. When taken over a long period of time (months to years), or when taken improperly, steroids can cause a myriad of side effects. But when asthma symptoms flare and are unresponsive to the nonsteroid medications, the benefit of steroids far outweighs the potential risks, especially for short-term use. For difficult-to-manage asthma, steroids can be a miraculous medication. For these important reasons all asthma patients should be aware of steroids and understand their proper use.

What Are Steroids? Steroids used in the treatment of asthma are man-made replications of a natural product of the adrenal glands. The adrenal glands are located just above the kidneys. The steroids produced by the adrenal glands serve three principal actions: (a) regulation of the body's salt, so that sodium is retained by the body and potassium is excreted—this favors salt and fluid retention, both of which are necessary for our body to function properly; (b) reduction of inflammation—it is this function which synthetic steroids presumably bring to asthma management; and (c) action in both males and females as a weak male hormone. In addition, steroids affect the way the body handles carbohydrates, proteins, and fats. Also, increased steroid production is one of the body's normal protective reactions to physical stress.

In view of the above, it is clear that steroids normally produced by the adrenal glands have a wide-ranging impact on the body. When synthetic steroids are administered over a prolonged period of time to manage asthma, thereby exposing the body to additional steroids, it is no wonder that the resulting side effects have impact on so many of the body's functions.

What Steroids Are Not. Steroids used for asthma management are not the same as steroids used by weight lifters for the purpose of increasing muscle mass. Steroids used by weight lifters are termed anabolic steroids. They are male hormones that are a product of the testes, not the adrenal gland.

How Do Steroids Work in Asthma? Over the years it has become evident that steroids are an effective asthma medication. Although the exact mechanism of how steroids work in managing asthma is still not clear-cut, it is known that steroids help to reduce inflammation within the airways of the asthma patient. In addition, steroids seem to allow other asthma medications to work better when asthma is out of control.

Steroid Production by the Body. You need to understand how the body produces steroids, so that you can appreciate the importance of taking steroids in as ideal a manner as possible.

A portion of the brain called the pituitary gland releases a chemical called ACTH (adrenocorticotropic hormone). ACTH stimulates the adrenal glands to release steroids. The brain's release of ACTH signals the adrenal glands to increase steroid production. In medical terms this pathway is referred to as the hypothalamic-pituitary-adrenal axis (HPA axis), as the pituitary gland is itself controlled by another portion of the brain called the hypothalamus (see Figure 3-3).

The brain's release of ACTH is also controlled by a "feedback loop." This means that the brain, before releasing ACTH, determines the amount of adrenal steroid already present in the circulation. When the level of circulating adrenal steroids is high, the brain identifies this and the ACTH level drops, resulting in no further release of steroid from the adrenal glands. Conversely, when the level of adrenal steroids in circulation is low, the brain senses this and the ACTH level increases, resulting in increased steroid release.

Steroids Are Normally Released in the Early Morning Hours. The brain releases ACTH, thus stimulating steroid production, in a daily cycle, with most of the adrenal

Normal Steroid Release   The Effect of Taking Steroid Medication

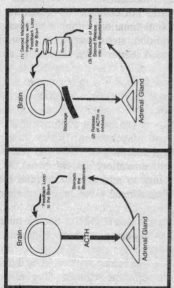

LEFT: The anterior pituitary gland in the brain releases a hormone called ACTH. ACTH stimulates the adrenal gland to release steroids into the bloodstream. Through a "feedback loop," the brain determines the amount of adrenal steroid in the bloodstream. When the steroid level is high, the brain does not release ACTH. When the steroid level is low, the brain releases ACTH to stimulate steroid production. This normally occurs in a cyclic pattern, with the greatest amount of steroid released in the early morning. RIGHT: Steroid medications interfere with normal steroid release from the adrenal gland. The brain detects the presence of the additional steroid in the bloodstream, and stops releasing ACTH early in the morning as it normally would. As a result, the adrenal gland's normal cyclic release of steroid is suppressed.

Figure 3-3.

steroid released in the early morning hours. The steroid level gradually decreases during the day, with the lowest level at midnight. This pattern correlates with our normal sleep pattern. Thus, if someone sleeps during the day and works during the evening, the pattern would be reversed. In addition to this daily steroid pattern, steroid release is increased during times of stress as a protective mechanism for the body.

The Effect of Oral Steroid Medications on the Body's Normal Steroid Production. When steroids are used in an asthma treatment plan, the presence of these additional steroids in the circulation indicates to the brain that no further steroid production is necessary. If oral steroid administration continues on a daily basis for months to years, the adrenal glands may lose their ability to respond to ACTH, and normal rhythmic steroid production is reduced or ceases. In fact, the adrenal glands can actually wither away because of nonuse (atrophy) and therefore remain nonfunctional once steroid medications are no longer taken. In this case, patients may have "adrenal insufficiency." Fortunately, for most patients, when oral steroids are discontinued, the adrenal glands are able to recover and resume normal steroid production with time, regardless of the length of time of steroid use.

Suppression of the adrenal glands puts asthma patients at risk in circumstances when increased adrenal secretion of steroids is needed, such as during the stress of surgery or infections. Adrenal insufficiency can lead to steroid withdrawal symptoms such as muscle and joint achiness, fatigue, weakness, and fever if oral steroids are suddenly discontinued. This occurs because the body has learned to rely on the steroid medication instead of producing steroids as it normally would. Therefore, you should never suddenly stop taking oral steroids on your own.

Steroid Side Effects. Side effects resulting from long-term oral steroid use are listed in Table 3–15. Side effects occur as a result of the body's prolonged exposure to extra steroids. The risk of developing steroid side effects depends on the length of time you take steroids and the amount which you

Some Potential Steroid Side Effects

1. Cataracts

2. Osteoporosis

3. Fullness of the face

4. Weight gain

5. Change in fat distribution ("buffalo hump")

6. High blood pressure

7. Increased blood sugar

8. Susceptibility to bruises

9. Altered growth (in children)

10. Muscle weakness

11. Skin changes: acne, thinning of the skin

12. Hair growth (especially on cheeks of females)

13. Decreased resistance to infection

14. Salt and fluid retention

15. Changes in mood

16. Suppression of normal steroid production

17. Risk of ulcer (debatable)

Table 3–15

take. As mentioned previously, steroids have an impact on many body functions, thereby explaining the wide range of potential side effects. One is suppression of normal steroid production as discussed above. The most serious consequences of long-term steroid use are weakening of the bones (osteoporosis) and growth retardation in young children.

These two side effects are usually irreversible. Cataracts are another common complication of long-term steroid therapy. Changes such as roundness of the face, development of facial hair, weight gain, elevation of the blood sugar and blood pressure, and swelling of the legs (edema) often improve if steroids can be reduced or discontinued. Be aware that even short-term steroid use can lead to weight gain caused by increased appetite as well as salt and water retention. An extensive review of current management approaches to steroid side effects is presented in Chapter 19.

Steroids Should Be Taken as Ideally as Possible. The key factors that influence the extent of adrenal gland suppression and the risk of steroid side effects with routine oral steroid use include: (a) the steroid agent chosen, (b) the time of day when steroids are taken, (c) the amount of steroids taken, and (d) the length of the treatment period. Oral steroids are used most safely under certain conditions: (a) if shorter-acting steroids are taken in preference to longer-acting products, (b) if single early morning steroid dosing (which mimics the body's normal steroid secretion pattern) is used, preferably every other day, as opposed to multiple doses taken during the day, and (c) if oral steroids are used for the shortest possible treatment period. Each of these factors is discussed in greater detail in the section on oral steroids later in this chapter.

CONCERN FOR STEROID SIDE EFFECTS AND ADRENAL FUNCTION SHOULD NOT INFLUENCE THE DECISION TO INITIATE STEROIDS DURING AN ACUTE, DIFFICULT-TO-MANAGE ASTHMA FLARE. SHORT COURSES OF STEROIDS, EVEN IN HIGH DOSES, CAN BE USED WITH LITTLE RISK OF LONG-TERM ADRENAL GLAND SUPPRESSION AND STEROID SIDE EFFECTS.

Short-Term Steroid Use. Steroids are given if asthma symptoms are out of control and nonsteroid medications have proven ineffective. It would be an error to withhold steroids in an acute, difficult-to-manage asthma attack. *THE RISK WITH STEROIDS, EVEN IN HIGH DOSES, IS NOT WITH OCCASIONAL SHORT-TERM USE BUT RATHER WITH*

THEIR LONG-TERM USE. This is a critical point. There-fore, if your doctor suggests a short course of steroids, you should understand that the risk is minimal. It is a myth that once steroids are started, you will always need steroids and become forever dependent on them. Steroids can be lifesaving when your asthma symptoms are truly severe. They should be administered early in an acute attack, as they take from four to six hours to work.

Routine Steroid Use. In view of their potential side ef-fects, oral steroids used in a routine manner should be the last alternative in any asthma program. Before your doctor concludes that you need routine long-term steroids, he should be certain that the dose and method of use of your current nonsteriod medications are correct. Your peak theophylline level should be checked to be certain that you are taking the right amount of theophylline. In addition, other asthma med-ications that do not contain steroids should be tried. If your doctor decides that you need steroids on a regular basis to keep your airways open, it is essential that you take them in the most ideal way possible. Your doctor should frequently reassess your need for routine steroids to see if steroids re-main necessary.

Steroid Choices. Steroids are available in both inhaled and oral preparations. The inhaled preparations have the advan-tage of being ''site specific''—that is, they act directly at the site of the problem (the airways), and thus have little effect on the rest of the body. Oral steroids, on the other hand, must be swallowed and thus have greater access to the entire body and a greater chance of leading to side effects. However, if your asthma can be well managed by using oral steroids every other day as a single early morning dose, the incidence of steroid side effects is far less than if you use oral steroids daily or twice daily. As a matter of fact, an argument can be made that low-dose oral steroids taken every other day as a single morning dose are as safe as using inhaled steroids.

Inhaled Steroids. The inhaled steroid preparations cur-rently available include beclomethasone (Vanceril and

Beclovent), flunisolide (AeroBid), and triamcinolone (Azmacort). The first steroid agent to be considered in a routine asthma program is often an inhaled product, on the basis of its site specificity and lesser risk of steroid side effects. These inhalers are typically used in dosage ranges of two to four puffs two to four times a day, but they can be used more frequently. Proper inhaler technique is essential. The technique previously described for inhaled bronchodilators is also used for inhaled steroids (see page 68). Frequently, inhaled steroids are used after using an inhaled bronchodilator to open the airways and allow the steroid better penetration into the airways. It must be emphasized that inhaled steroids are preventative medications. They do not immediately relieve your asthma symptoms. However, they will help stabilize and gradually even out your asthma symptoms, ultimately resulting in fewer asthma flares.

Inhaled Steroids Can Replace or Help Reduce Oral Steroids. The addition of inhaled steroids to an asthma management plan can often reduce the asthma patient's oral steroid requirement. Many patients are able to discontinue oral steroids altogether. Any reduction of oral steroids that can be accomplished with the addition of inhaled steroids is worthwhile, as this will usually allow normal adrenal gland function to resume and the risk of steroid side effects to decrease. Reduction of the oral steroid dose must be made gradually. Careful observation by your doctor of your spirometry (breathing test) results is an important aid to sound decision-making. Above all, never change your steroid dose without first consulting your doctor.

Oral Steroids May Still Be Necessary. If your treatment plan includes inhaled steroids and your asthma begins to flare, notify your doctor early as a short course of oral steroids may be necessary. The inhaled steroids you normally take may not be sufficient to control a difficult asthma flare. Inhaled steroids are a preventative medication when used routinely and should never be viewed as an alternative to oral steroids for controlling an asthma flare.

Inhaler Technique Is Important. Be certain that you are using the inhaler correctly. The technique is the same as that for the bronchodilating inhalers (see Figure 3-3). If your doctor suggests using two puffs at a time of your steroid inhaler, this means two separate inhalation maneuvers, one for each puff. Common mistakes made by some patients include: (a) spraying both puffs directly into the mouth at the same time, (b) failing to inhale at the same time as the inhaler is activated, and (c) placing the inhaler directly into the mouth (rather than a few inches away) so that the inhaled medication simply splashes against the back of the throat. Avoid these mistakes to get the fullest benefit from your inhaled steroids.

Inhaled Steroids Are Not for Children Under Five. Steroids for inhalation are available only in the form of spray-type inhalers. They are not available in liquid form for inhalation with the use of a nebulizer. Therefore, you must be able to master proper inhaler technique in order to use inhaled steroids. Most children under the age of five are unable to use an inhaler properly and thus are not able to use inhaled steroids. However, inhalation chambers, such as InspirEase and Inhalaid, may allow young children to use inhaled steroids as an alternative to oral steroids for long-term use.

Thrush, the Major Side Effect of Inhaled Steroids. The major side effect of inhaled steroids is thrush, a yeast infection involving the back of the throat. If thrush is present, a whitish film can be seen around the tonsil area and the back of the throat. Although thrush can cause your throat to be irritated, you may have thrush and be free of any symptoms. If you notice any signs of thrush you should notify your doctor. Since thrush is sometimes an early clue of underlying diabetes, your doctor should explore this possibility if thrush persists.

Careful review of your inhaler technique is important, as incorrect use of the inhaler can lead to thrush by coating the back of the throat with steroid, as opposed to aerosolizing the steroid into the lungs. A specially designed spacing device is often helpful in such a case, since it increases the distance from the inhaler to the back of the throat and thus allows the steroid to become better aerosolized (see page 70).

A case of thrush can sometimes be cleared up by reducing the dose of inhaled steroid, if possible. Also, a simple way of reducing the chance of developing thrush is to rinse your mouth and gargle with warm water after using the inhaler to remove any medication remaining in the throat. Once thrush develops, nystatin (Mycostatin) mouthwash is usually sufficient to keep it under control. The typical dose of Mycostatin mouthwash is 1 teaspoon (5 cc) to swirl, gargle, and spit out after using your inhaler. Often just a week's worth of therapy is sufficient.

No Long-Term Side Effects Clearly Linked to Inhaled Steroids to Date. When the dosage of inhaled steroids is kept within the recommended range, the risk of suppression of the body's normal steroid production is small and the chance of serious steroid side effects is significantly less than with oral steroids, although still possible. However, the long-term effect on the throat of inhaling steroids is still unknown.

Oral Steroids. Because of their risk of side effects with long-term use, oral steroids should be used on a routine basis only when nothing else will control your asthma. For most asthma patients, steroids along with theophylline and inhaled or oral Adrenalin-like bronchodilators can help keep asthma symptoms under control. However, the potential for steroid side effects emphasizes the importance of using oral steroids in as ideal a manner as possible. Close follow-up with your doctor with a watchful eye toward the potential for steroid reduction is important. You should be aware of the intended benefit and possible risks of long-term use of oral steroids.

Short-Acting Steroids Are Preferable. Oral steroids are available in several different forms, as shown in Table 3–16. The short- and intermediate-acting steroids are the most appropriate for treating asthma. Shorter-acting steroids include prednisone, prednisolone, and methylprednisolone (Medrol). Methylprednisolone causes less salt retention than prednisone

Best Choices of Oral Steroid Agents for Asthma Care (Alphabetically):

Shorter-Acting
- Methylprednisolone (Medrol)
- Prednisolone
- Prednisone

Oral Steroids Best Avoided (If Possible) for Asthma Care:

Longer-Acting
- Dexamethasone (Decadron)
- Triamcinolone (Aristocort)

Table 3–16

and is therefore a better choice for patients with heart or blood pressure problems. Longer-acting products such as dexamethasone or triamcinolone, which can be given orally or as an intramuscular injection, should not be used for routine asthma care because they will suppress the hypothalamic-pituitary-adrenal axis more than the shorter-acting products do. The shorter-acting products allow the pathway between the brain and the adrenal gland to recover so that normal steroid production can continue. In addition, the longer-acting steroids are more potent and carry a greater risk of side effects. If you are now using one of the longer-acting steroids, an important first step toward reducing your chances of steroid side effects is to ask your doctor if you can substitute one of the shorter-acting steroids.

The Importance of Taking Oral Steroids Early in the Morning.

As previously discussed, steroids are secreted by the adrenal glands primarily in the early morning hours. Any additional steroids that you routinely need to control your asthma should be taken early in the morning when the body is secreting its own steroid. The brain will send its routine message that the adrenal glands should continue normal steroid production, and the risk of adrenal gland suppression will be reduced.

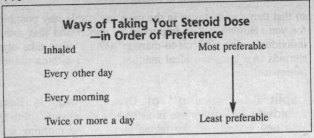

Table 3-17

Steroids Are Not to Be Taken Randomly During the Day.

If oral steroids are taken randomly during the day, especially during times when the body does not normally put out steroids, the message from the brain to the adrenal glands is that routine steroid production early in the morning is no longer necessary, as the body has plenty of steroids. For this reason oral steroids for asthma management should, if at all possible, be taken in the early morning hours.

"Alternate Day Dosing"—The Ideal Way of Taking Oral Steroids.

Use of oral steroids every other day is by far the preferable way of taking oral steroids. Alternate day dosing allows sufficient time between steroid doses for the adrenal glands to recover so that they can work normally. The risk of side effects is far less when oral steroids are taken in this manner. Many doctors feel that the small amount of oral steroids taken on an alternate day dosing schedule is as safe as using an inhaled steroid preparation. In addition, it is far more convenient to remember to take a pill every other morning than it is to use an inhaler four times a day every day. The choice between alternate day oral steroids and inhaled steroids is a matter of personal preference debated among doctors. Many doctors still favor the inhaled steroids because of their ability to work directly at the site of the problem (the airways) despite the inconvenience.

Table 3-17 lists my preferences for administering oral steroids. An effort should be made from time to time to reassess the dosage and the manner in which you take oral steroids,

so that they can be taken in the most preferable way possible
for you. However, it is important to understand that some
individuals with difficult-to-manage asthma must take oral
steroids in a less than ideal manner, as their asthma cannot
otherwise be controlled.

**"Split Daily Dosing" of Oral Steroids Is Best
Avoided.** For routine use in asthma management, splitting
your oral steroid dose by taking some in the morning and
some later in the day carries the greatest risk of steroid side
effects and adrenal suppression. You should ask your doctor
whether you are a candidate for taking your steroids as a
single morning dose rather than splitting the dose during the
day. A larger dose of steroid taken all at once in the early
morning is probably less suppressive of normal steroid production than small doses taken throughout the day. Any
changes in your steroid dose should first be reviewed with
your doctor, as there are some patients who have such frequent and severe asthma symptoms that they are unable to be
managed with less frequent steroid scheduling.

Steroid Dosages. There are no fixed rules for the correct
dosage of oral steroids in asthma management. Your doctor
will determine how much steroid you need based on your
breathing test and the status of your asthma. Fine-tuning of
your steroid requirement will take place as your doctor follows your progress.

It is important to contact your doctor early during an acute
flare of asthma. A few large doses of oral steroid taken early
during an acute flare may help to avert severe prolonged
asthma symptoms. Steroids may be administered several times
during the day in order to maximize their effects. However,
as soon as the acute attack is under control, the dose is often
consolidated to a single morning dose and then tapered to the
minimal amount necessary to keep the symptoms under control. For a patient who does not require routine steroids, oral
steroids can be added for a few days if asthma symptoms are
severe, and then often be discontinued. For patients who routinely require oral steroids, asthma attacks are often best
managed by increasing (boosting) the steroid dose to get the

symptoms under control, and then gradually tapering the dose to the minimal amount necessary to keep the symptoms under control. In the emergency room, high doses of steroids are administered early in the course of a difficult asthma episode. **REMEMBER:** *IT TAKES FROM FOUR TO SIX HOURS FOR STEROIDS TO WORK, SO THEY ARE BEST GIVEN EARLY IN AN ACUTE ASTHMA FLARE.*

Steroid Dosage for the Acute Flare. Typical doses of oral steroid used for acute asthma flares in adults are 30 to 60 milligrams of prednisone. This dose is often continued for 3 days and then gradually reduced. For small children, a rule of thumb is to administer daily 2 milligrams of oral steroid for each kilogram of the child's weight, with the medication often divided during the day. However, steroid dosing must be determined by the physician in each individual case. Short-term dosing is generally not as critical as determining the dose for long-term use. Above all, see your doctor if steroids have been added or increased so that appropriate adjustments in your asthma program can be made.

Steroid Dosing in Status Asthmaticus. When asthma symptoms are out of control and unresponsive to Adrenalin and other nonsteroid medications, this is called status asthmaticus. Large intravenous steroid doses are often administered at frequent intervals in the hope of controlling the symptoms. Typical adult doses of steroids range from 100 to 150 milligrams of hydrocortisone (Solu-Cortef), or from 30 to 250 milligrams of methylprednisolone (Solu-Medrol). Intravenous steroids are usually given at 4- to 6-hour intervals until the symptoms are under better control. As stated previously, there is little concern for side effects from short-term use of steroids, even at high doses. It is for this reason that doctors use large doses of steroid for status asthmaticus. There are no fixed rules concerning tapering of steroid dosages once status asthmaticus begins to improve; reduction of the steroid dose is done on an individual basis, with the doctor closely assessing the patient's progress.

Steroid Dosing in Children. The guidelines for steroid

use in children are similar to those for adults, except for dosages. In the emergency situation, steroids should be administered early in a difficult asthma flare if nonsteroid medications fail to provide relief. In such a situation, it would be a mistake to withhold steroids simply because the patient is a child. For routine use, children who fail to respond to nonsteroid medications may well be candidates for routine steroids.

The dose of steroid is determined by the doctor on the basis of the child's age, size, and severity of symptoms. In an acute setting the dose is often split, with steroid taken several times during the day. This is fine for a short period of use. The concern with long-term steroid use by children is for the potential of growth retardation. Thus, if steroids must be taken on a routine basis by children, it is especially important that the steroids be administered properly (see page 110).

Chronic Dosing of Oral Steroids. There are no fixed rules about long-term dosing of oral steroids other than to use the minimal amount necessary to control asthma symptoms. The appropriate dose is determined by your doctor with careful observation over time. Certainly, steroids should be taken in as ideal a manner as possible to reduce the risk of steroid side effects. Emphasis should be placed on (a) utilizing a short-acting steroid preparation, (b) taking the smallest dose possible, (c) using steroid only in the early morning hours, if possible, and (d) using steroid on an alternate day schedule, if possible.

Steroids Are Best Taken with Food. Oral steroids can irritate the stomach and therefore should be taken with food, which will serve as a buffer to reduce the irritation. It is thought that oral steroids can also contribute to the development of ulcers, although this point is controversial among doctors. If you have a tendency to develop ulcers or a tendency to bleed from your gastrointestinal tract, you should mention this to your doctor.

Steroid Dose Must Be Increased in Times of Stress. Patients on long-term steroid therapy will require supplemental doses of steroids during physically stressful situations such as surgery or infections. As a precaution, patients who have needed oral steroids during the past year should also be given supplemental steroids with surgery. The reason for this is that the body normally puts out more steroids in response to stress to allow the body to handle the stress better. However, in a patient who routinely takes oral steroids for asthma management, normal adrenal gland production of steroid is suppressed; the body is then unable to put out additional steroids in times of stress.

The use of supplemental steroids in times of stress is critical. This point is well known to doctors, but is important for you to remember if you are away from your doctor and require surgery or develop an infection. If you have frequently used oral steroids during the past year, you should carry a card in your wallet or wear a Medi-Alert bracelet that indicates this.

Reduction in Steroid Use. Steroid dosing should be reassessed routinely by your doctor. The dose of steroid for patients on routine oral steroid therapy can sometimes be reduced during symptom-free intervals. Because your body has become accustomed to taking in additional steroids, it is possible to experience some side effects as the dose of oral steroids is reduced. These may include fatigue and achiness of the joints. For this reason the dose should be reduced gradually in someone who has taken steroids for a prolonged period. If you experience any unusual symptoms as your oral steroid dose is reduced, notify your doctor. It may be necessary to temporarily increase your steroid dose until you are feeling better and then to reduce your steroid dose more slowly.

Rules to be Followed When Taking Steroids. Rules that should be followed when using steroids include: (a) Take the steroids at the prescribed time and in the prescribed amount—do not alter the dose on your own. (b) Never stop your steroids on your own. (c) Be sure that all your doctors (including your dentist) know that you are taking steroids. (d) Remember that your steroid dose should be increased during

Steroids—Essential Points

- Steroids should be the last medication added to a **routine** asthma program because of concern for long-term side effects. For an **acute** asthma flare which does not respond to your routine medications, steroids are essential and may be lifesaving.

- **It would be a mistake to refuse to take steroids during an acute, difficult-to-manage asthma attack.** Steroids should be taken early during an acute attack because there is a 4–6 hour delay before steroids work.

Table 3–18

times of stress—carry this reminder with you on a Medi-Alert bracelet or in your wallet.

Steroids should be used to manage asthma only if they are necessary. The essential points in this regard are summarized in Table 3–18. If steroids are needed, they should be used as ideally as possible to reduce the potential of side effects.

QUESTIONS

1. I've heard from friends what steroids can do to you. I'll never take them. Don't you agree?

No. Steroids can be a potentially lifesaving medication during a difficult-to-manage asthma flare. It would be a mistake to refuse to take them out of fear of side effects or dependency, if your doctor or an emergency room doctor thinks you need them to control an asthma flare. Side effects such as increased blood sugar, fluid retention, and weight gain, which at times are associated with the short-term use of steroids, are usually transient and easily managed. The potentially serious side effects from steroids are usually associated only with their long-term use.

2. It appears that I need steroids on a routine basis to control my asthma. Are there any alternatives?

Certainly every alternative should be tried prior to using steroids on a long-term basis. Your current medication program should be carefully reviewed. Worthwhile questions include: (a) Has your dose of theophylline been checked at the appropriate time (peak or trough) to be certain that you are receiving the ideal dose? (b) Do you use your inhaler(s) properly and at the correct times? (c) Have nonsteroid alternatives such as cromolyn sodium and oral Adrenalin-like bronchodilators been tried? If each of these alternatives has been considered and your asthma is still difficult to manage, there may not be an alternative to the use of steroids.

Your effort should then be directed to asking if you are using steroids in as ideal a manner as possible to lessen the risk of side effects. The most preferable choices would be to use either inhaled steroids or steroids taken every other day in the early morning hours. If your asthma cannot be controlled with alternate day steroids, then a single early morning steroid dose is the next most preferable means of steroid administration. Split daily dosing of steroids (taking some in the morning and some later in the day) should be avoided if possible, except during acute worsening of your asthma, because there is an increased risk of side effects when steroids are taken in this manner for the long term. The use of long-acting steroids, such as dexamethasone or triamcinolone, also increases the risk of steroid side effects and should be avoided.

3. Why do steroid side effects occur?

Steroid side effects are the result of the body's overexposure to steroids. The body normally produces steroids in the adrenal glands. Steroids administered for asthma management are synthetic replications of these adrenal steroids. The steroids produced in the adrenal glands have impact on many functions of the body, thereby explaining why overexposure to steroids results in such a myriad of side effects (see Chapter 19).

4. Will steroids build up my muscles, like a weight lifter's?

No. Steroids taken by weight lifters are male testicular hormones. Steroids used in asthma management are adrenal hormones, and tend to weaken the muscles rather than strengthen them when used over a long period of time.

5. Why is it important that I take additional steroids when I'm in a physically stressful situation?

If you routinely take steroids or have taken steroids intermittently during the past year, it is possible that your adrenal gland is suppressed and unable to secrete additional steroids as it normally would during times of stress. Therefore, if you require surgery or have a serious infection, supplemental steroids may be a necessity. You should carry a Medi-Alert bracelet or a card in your wallet indicating that you take steroids routinely or have needed steroids during the past year, to provide this information in the event that you become unconscious during an emergency.

6. My doctor has prescribed steroids to manage my asthma and I've been taking them routinely for the past six months. Does this mean that I will always need steroids?

There is no definitive answer to your question. Your doctor should reassess the status of your asthma frequently to determine whether your steroid requirement has changed. It is important to use as little oral steroid as is necessary to control your asthma symptoms. Your doctor, not you, must determine the steroid dose. A larger dose of steroid taken every other day in the early morning is usually associated with less steroid side effects than even a much smaller dose taken every day. Therefore, as a first step, review with your doctor whether your asthma can be controlled with alternate day steroids. The addition of inhaled steroids, if not already being used, can also assist in lowering the steroid dose still further. Some patients are able to discontinue use of oral steroids if inhaled steroids are added to their program.

Periodic reassessment of the dosing and means of administration of the nonsteroid medications is also important. Steroid dose adjustments are typically made slowly if you have been using steroids for a while, to avoid withdrawal symptoms such as fatigue and achiness of the joints.

7. I get a sore throat when I use my steroid inhaler. Should I continue to use it?

Yes. First you should ask your doctor to observe your inhaler technique. The steroid in the inhaler can irritate the throat, especially if your inhaler technique is less than ideal. By holding the inhaler away from your mouth when you use it, you increase the likelihood that the steroid will become properly aerosolized and enter your lungs, as opposed to hitting the back of your throat. Rinse your mouth with water after using inhaled steroids to remove any of the medication that might remain. If you have thrush, a condition in which whitish patches appear on the back of the throat, your doctor will prescribe nystatin (Mycostatin) mouthwash for use after the inhaled steroid. With time, the nystatin will usually reduce the irritation.

8. I needed steroids for my last asthma flare. My face got swollen and I gained weight, so I stopped the steroids. Did I do the right thing?

No. Steroid dosages and reduction schedules should be determined by your doctor. The side effects you describe are no doubt troublesome, but they are usually reversible once you are no longer taking steroids. Remember that the reason you needed steroids in the first place was to be able to breathe. You should not simply stop the steroids without your doctor's approval, as your asthma may again flare. However, you can ask your doctor to reassess your steroid requirement in light of your current breathing status and any side effects you may have developed.

9. My five-year-old has difficult-to-manage asthma. His attacks are severe at times. I have always resisted the use of steroids, as steroids for a child so young scare me. Don't you agree?

I agree that oral steroids used on a regular basis should be the last alternative for all patients, especially for a five-year-old child. Every alternative to the routine use of oral steroids should be considered. However, the use of oral steroids for a difficult-to-manage asthma attack presents a different situation. The short-term use of oral steroids for asthma symptoms that are out of control can be a potentially lifesaving decision. In this situation, the age of the patient makes no difference, as the goal is to open the airways, reduce inflammation of the airways, and allow free breathing.

10. If I forget to take my steroids when I am supposed to at 7:00 A.M., should I take them as soon as I remember or should I take them the next day at 7:00 A.M.?

You should take your steroid dose as soon as you remember. If your doctor has prescribed routine steroids for you, this indicates that you need steroids to keep your airways open. If you do not take them, your asthma might begin to flare. Therefore, you should not skip a day unless you were instructed to do so by your doctor. The logic behind the 7:00 A.M. dosing schedule is that this is close to the time when the body normally secretes its own steroids. The steroids you take for your asthma are not "noticed" as much by the brain if you mimic the adrenal gland's own steroid secretion time by taking your steroids in the early morning. Steroids taken at times other than the early morning hours have a greater chance of suppressing the body's normal steroid production. Although risk of adrenal gland suppression is somewhat greater when the forgotten dose is taken later in the day, it is important above all else that your normal steroid dose be taken to prevent asthma symptoms from developing.

11. If I suddenly stopped taking my routine oral steroids, would I die?

If routine oral steroids have been necessary for several years to manage asthma and are abruptly discontinued, the greatest risk is that of a severe, potentially life-threatening asthma attack. In addition, there are potential withdrawal symptoms if steroids are stopped abruptly, which can include fatigue, achiness in the legs or stomach, nausea, and vomiting. In rare instances, steroid withdrawal which is too abrupt can over a period of time lead to death. Your doctor should periodically reassess your need for routine daily steroids, but you should never discontinue steroids on your own.

12. If I start getting steroid side effects, should I stop taking steroids?

Presumably you have been taking steroids because there is no alternative. Although your need for long-term oral steroids should have been frequently reassessed over the years, this is a good time to make certain that your airways cannot be kept open except with the use of routine oral steroids. Discuss this issue with your doctor. If steroids are necessary to keep your airways open, this will outweigh the unfortunate occurrence of steroid side effects.

SUMMARY: STEROIDS

1. The steroid medications used in asthma management are man-made replications of the anti-inflammatory hormones of the adrenal gland.

2. Steroids clearly are beneficial in asthma management. However, the benefit achieved with oral steroids must be weighed against the potential risks associated with long-term steroid use.

3. If oral steroids are needed on a routine basis to keep asthma under control, using them under ideal conditions can reduce the risk of developing side effects. The most preferable way to use oral steroids includes: (a) use of an early morning dosage schedule, preferably every other day, as opposed to taking steroids several times during the day; (b) use of shorter-acting steroid preparations such as prednisone, prednisolone, or methylprednisolone, as opposed to longer-acting agents such as injected or oral dexamethasone or triamcinolone; and (c) use of the smallest amount of steroids needed to control asthma symptoms, taken as infrequently as possible.

4. Short courses of oral steroids, even in high doses, can be used with little risk of long-term adrenal gland suppression and steroid side effects. The risk with oral ste-

roids, even in high doses, is not with occasional short-term use but rather with their long-term use.

5. Oral steroids should be started early in severe asthma episodes that are unresponsive to the nonsteroid medications, as steroids take four to six hours to work. For difficult-to-manage asthma, steroids can be a lifesaving medication.

6. For patients who take oral steroids on a routine basis or have taken steroids intermittently during the past year, supplemental steroids must be taken in times of stress (such as surgery or a serious infection or accident). Carry a card in your wallet or wear a Medi-Alert bracelet if you have used steroids routinely or intermittently during the past year.

7. Steroid side effects are a result of prolonged exposure to steroid medication. Table 3–15 and Chapter 19 review potential side effects of steroids.

8. Inhaled steroids offer the advantage of acting directly at the site of the problem (the airways) with less absorption of steroid into the body. Often, the oral steroid dose can be reduced or discontinued with the addition of inhaled steroids. Inhaled steroids are preventative agents intended for routine use—they do not offer immediate relief of your asthma symptoms.

9. Inhaled steroids in conventional dosages carry only a small risk of steroid side effects. The major side effect of inhaled steroid use is thrush, a yeast infection resulting in whitish patches on the tongue and the back of the throat. Thrush is prevented by rinsing your mouth with water after inhaler use, reducing the dose of inhaled steroids, and using nystatin (Mycostatin) mouthwash, if necessary.

10. Steroids should be taken in the prescribed amount and at the prescribed time. Any changes in the dose or timing should be made only by your doctor. Steroids should be

used only if necessary; if they are needed, they should be used properly to reduce the potential of side effects.

E. MISCELLANEOUS MEDICATIONS

Atropine and Atropinelike Medications. Atropine is an effective bronchodilator. It works by partially blocking the vagus nerve, which controls the normal, slightly constrictive tone of the airways, resulting in relaxation of the muscles surrounding the airways and, ultimately, opening of the airways. Although atropine offers the advantage of working differently than (yet compatibly with) theophylline, it has not been used extensively in the United States because of its airway drying effect (with concern for mucus plugging of the airways) and potential for side effects such as rapid heartbeat.

Atropine is used only as an inhaled medication in a nebulizer, in a similar fashion as one would use isoetharine or metaproterenol. It is now used only for difficult-to-manage asthma, and may be helpful in asthma patients who produce excessive mucus. Atropine is typically first tried in a hospital setting, to be certain of its effect on the patient's heart rate. Prolonged use of high dose atropine can cause dryness of the mouth, blurred vision, difficulty urinating (especially in older men), and even mental disturbances. Therefore, this medication should only be prescribed by a physician familiar with its use and complications. At times, atropine can be a very successful addition to an asthma program.

Newer atropinelike agents such as ipratropium bromide (SCH 1000 and Atrovent) offer the advantage of being free of the typical atropine side effects. Currently, these newer agents are unavailable for use in the United States. Ipratropium bromide is available in England as an inhaler. It is used in a dosage of one to two puffs three times a day. It opens the airways slowly but its effect can be long-lasting (up to four hours). Preliminary studies suggest that it may be useful in conjunction with (not as a replacement for) the other asthma medications. In addition, ipratropium may prove useful for individuals whose asthma is made worse by emotional upset. One explanation for this is that with emotional upset, the tone of the vagus nerve is increased, resulting in constriction of the airway. By reducing the tone of the airway, ipratropium may reduce asthma symptoms in this setting.

Atropine and the newer atropinelike medications are at present considered to be experimental medications, and have not been approved for use in the United States. Studies suggest that, with time, these medications will gain approval and have a place in asthma management for certain individuals.

Expectorants. The logic for the use of expectorants in asthma management is to thin the sticky mucus in the airways, making it easier to clear the mucus by coughing. However, it is controversial whether the currently available expectorants really accomplish this goal. Most doctors do not include expectorants in their asthma management plans.

Potassium iodide is the most commonly used expectorant. It has the disadvantage of potential side effects such as acne, increased salivation, and hives. In addition, the use of iodides can interfere with the body's normal production of thyroid hormones, resulting in low thyroid function and goiters (enlargement of the thyroid gland). Low thyroid function can cause symptoms such as weakness and fatigue; in children it can have impact on proper growth and development. In view of their small chance of a beneficial effect and their potential risk of side effects, iodide expectorants should be used sparingly. In general, they are best avoided by children, especially for long-term use. Iodides should be avoided during pregnancy and by women who are breast-feeding.

Like potassium iodide, guaifenesin is found in a number of asthma products. Its usefulness is controversial. Guaifenesin is thought to increase the output of fluid from the respiratory tract. This fluid is relatively thin and helps to liquefy the thick mucus secretions found in the airways of asthma patients, ultimately making it easier to clear these secretions by coughing. However, guaifenesin can also serve as an irritant to the airways and, in rare instances, can trigger coughing on its own. Some theophylline combination products contain guaifenesin as one of the ingredients. As previously discussed, these combination products have fallen into disfavor, since it is not possible to increase the dosage of theophylline when necessary without also increasing the other ingredients, which are usually not required in additional amounts (see page 86).

Antihistamines. Antihistamines are used primarily to treat symptoms of hay fever including nasal itchiness, sneezing, and runny nose. In general, antihistamines are not effective in opening the airways and relieving asthma symptoms. This is somewhat surprising. As histamine is one of the chemical mediators released from the mast cell in allergic individuals during asthma flares, it would seem logical that a product that counteracts the effect of histamine would help to relieve asthma symptoms. The fact that there is an array of chemical mediators released, not just histamine, may explain why antihistamines do not seem to help open the airways. However, it is becoming increasingly clear in asthma management that secretions in the upper airway (the nose, throat, and sinuses) can have impact on the lower airway (the breathing tubes) (see Chapter 17). Often asthma symptoms can be more easily managed if nasal and sinus problems are under better control. Therefore, for some individuals with asthma, antihistamines that are used to improve nasal symptoms may help to improve chest symptoms.

Most package labels for antihistamines contain warnings about the use of antihistamines by asthma patients. The concern is that airway drying may worsen asthma symptoms by making secretions such as mucus plugs more difficult to clear. For some patients this may be the case, but for most asthma patients, antihistamines can be used under their doctors' supervision with little worry. Certainly it is important to notify your doctor if you notice that the use of antihistamines is making your asthma worse, or causing you to become overly sleepy. Often antihistamines are used in combination with decongestants (see below). Commonly used antihistamine preparations include over-the-counter products such as Chlor-Trimeton, Drixoral, Actifed, and Triaminic, and prescription items such as Deconamine, Tavist, Trinalin, Polaramine, Isoclor, Fedahist, and Kronafed-A Jr. The frequently used product diphenhydramine (Benadryl) is more appropriate for allergic reactions such as hives or swelling than for nasal symptoms.

A recent addition to the spectrum of antihistamines is the

medication terfenedine (Seldane), available by prescription. Unlike most other antihistamines, it does not usually cause drowsiness.

Decongestants. Decongestants such as pseudoephedrine (Sudafed and Novafed) and phenylpropanolamine (Propagest and Entex) can decrease stuffiness of the nose. Interestingly, they also can act as mild bronchodilators. The use of a decongestant is permissible during an asthma flare. Decongestants can cause nervousness, headache, and nausea (the same as the side effects of theophylline and the Adrenalin-like bronchodilators). Sometimes your doctor will have you discontinue use of a decongestant during an asthma flare if an oral Adrenalin-like bronchodilator is needed, with concern for the combined stimulant effect of these medications. Decongestants can help to reduce nasal congestion and the resulting pressure within the sinuses. As mentioned previously, improvement in problems of the nose, sinuses, and upper airway can also help to improve asthma symptoms.

Use of Troleandomycin (TaO) to Reduce Steroid Dose. In an attempt to reduce high dose steroid requirements when all other changes in the medication program prove unrewarding, consideration can be given to the use of troleandomycin, a medication which is similar to erythromycin. It is unknown just how TaO (pronounced "tay-oh") works to allow the steroid dose to be reduced. Yet it is clear that, when used properly, TaO can allow the steroid dose to be reduced to remarkably lower levels, even to alternate-day dosing. TaO appears to be effective only when used with the steroid preparation methylprednisolone (Medrol). The most important benefits seem to be that patients are able to exercise somewhat more freely and gain a greater sense of well-being. Side effects from TaO can include nausea, vomiting, severe changes in liver function tests, and, at times, a worsening of steroid side effects (although this point is controversial). Without question, a trial use of TaO should be performed only by a doctor who is experienced with this medication. TaO is certainly one of the last alternatives in attempting to reduce the steroid requirement.

SUMMARY: MISCELLANEOUS MEDICATIONS

1. Atropine is an effective bronchodilator for some patients but should be reserved for difficult asthma because of its potential side effects, such as rapid heart rate and drying of the airways.

2. Newer atropinelike medications such as ipratropium bromide (SCH 1000 and Atrovent) are free of the typical atropine side effects but as yet are not available for use in the United States.

3. Expectorants are of questionable value in asthma management but are sometimes used in the hope that they can help to thin mucus in the airways, making it easier to clear by coughing.

4. Antihistamines can be used by asthma patients for managing nasal secretions. The concern that antihistamines will dry the airways, thereby triggering asthma symptoms, only applies to a small percentage of asthma patients. Often the benefit of improving upper airway symptoms offsets the small risk that antihistamines will cause an asthma flare due to airway drying.

5. Decongestants can decrease nasal stuffiness and act as a mild bronchodilator. In contrast to antihistamines, decongestants are not sedating.

6. Troleandomycin (TaO) is an erythromycin-like medication that helps reduce the steroid requirements of asthma patients who require high daily doses of steroid to manage their asthma. TaO seems to be effective only with the steroid preparation methylprednisolone (Medrol). As TaO does carry a risk of side effects, it must be prescribed by a doctor familiar with its use. TaO is reserved for use as one of the last alternatives for patients with difficult asthma, who are already taking high daily doses of oral steroids.

F. NEW MEDICATIONS

The innovative work taking place today in asthma research constantly suggests new ideas that often can be translated into new approaches toward asthma treatment. Often, new medications offer only slight changes in medications already available. However, a slight change in chemical structure of a medication may free that medication of a troublesome side effect or make it act more directly on the lungs. Clearly, there is hope that the future will bring greater understanding of asthma and fresh approaches toward therapy. Some of the medications that may be available in the near future are presented in this section.

Adrenalin-Like Bronchodilators. As previously discussed, newer medications have been developed that are longer lasting and act more directly on the airways (with less effect on the heart) than Adrenalin. Examples of these products include albuterol and terbutaline, which are in widespread use. Products of this type still under investigation include fenoterol, carbuterol, and procaterol. Bitolterol (Tornalate) is now available. Time will tell if these newer products offer anything different than albuterol, which represents the current state of the art with regard to bronchodilating medications.

Albuterol solution for nebulizer use is not available as of this writing but is scheduled for release in the near future.

Medications Similar to Cromolyn Sodium. The usefulness of cromolyn sodium as a preventative medication has triggered research into new cromolynlike medications that may last longer and be more potent and can be taken orally. Many of these products are still in the stage of preliminary studies, so it is difficult to comment fairly on their potential usefulness.

One such product, ketotifen, which is used in other countries but is not yet approved for use in the United States, shows great promise as it offers the advantage of being an oral preparation taken twice a day. Early studies indicate that ketotifen takes several weeks to produce an effect, as opposed to cromolyn sodium, which can take just a few days. Ketotifen's chemical structure is similar to that of the antihistamine cyproheptadine (Periactin) and, like cyproheptadine, can cause sedation during its initial use. It has been suggested that ketotifen may allow patients on steroids to reduce their dosage, but this point has not been well established.

Another cromolynlike product, called lodoxamide, is also being studied. It is currently an experimental medication which can be used both orally and by inhalation. Preliminary testing revealed side effects when taken orally such as vomiting, headache, and the sensation of generalized body heat; it is possible that, when the proper dosage for this medication is worked out, these side effects may become less troublesome. Inhaled lodoxamide has been shown to be of benefit as a pretreatment before allergen exposure, with a duration of action of up to four hours. In the inhaled form, lodoxamide appears to be free of side effects.

Atropinelike Medications. Atropine has been shown to be an effective bronchodilator and is used by some asthma specialists for some patients. However, the major drawback of atropine is side effects such as an increased heart rate, dryness of the mouth, urinary retention, and transient visual changes. Ipratropium bromide (SCH 1000 and Atrovent) offers the advantage of atropinelike action but also offers the potential of being relatively free of the atropinelike side effects. This medication appears to have a slow onset of action but a long duration and its best use may be in combination with bronchodilating medications. Although it is not yet available in the United States, it offers the promise of providing an additional asthma medication choice to physicians.

Calcium Antagonists. In order for the mast cell to release its chemical mediators such as histamine, an influx of calcium is required into the cell. In addition, mucus gland secretion and the contraction of smooth muscles (such as the muscles surrounding the airways) also require calcium influx. This observation has directed research toward a group of medications that will prevent the movement of calcium into these cells and thereby interfere with these actions. An approach to asthma management using calcium antagonists is now under investigation. The currently available calcium antagonists (such as nifedipine and verapamil, which are used routinely for heart problems) have been shown to have some benefit in blocking exercise-induced and allergen-induced asthma in the laboratory. As reports on the success of these agents vary, and as research for newer calcium antagonists that are more specific to the lung is still in progress, calcium antagonists have not been suggested for routine use in asthma care.

SUMMARY: NEW MEDICATIONS

1. Asthma research constantly seeks fresh approaches to asthma therapy. Often, existing medications are modified slightly to develop new medications that act longer or are free of an undesirable side effect.

2. Some of the products currently under investigation include inhaled and oral Adrenalin-like bronchodilators (fenoterol, carbuterol, bitolterol, and procaterol), cromolynlike medications which can be taken orally as well as inhaled (ketotifen and lodoxamide), atropinelike bronchodilators (ipratropium bromide), and calcium antagonists (nifedipine and verapamil).

3. It is to be hoped that the future will bring a clearer understanding of the basic causes of asthma, so that asthma can in fact be cured, not just well managed.

◇ 4 ◇

General Measures

Patient Education Is Essential. Management of any chronic illness such as asthma requires a close working relationship between doctor and patient. You need to have confidence in your doctor and feel comfortable talking with him or her. Hopefully your doctor will provide you with reading material concerning asthma and your medication therapy. You should become familiar with all aspects of asthma care so that you can take an active role in keeping your symptoms under control.

Patients who are experiencing asthma symptoms are often quite nervous. This is not abnormal, as shortness of breath and uncontrollable coughing and wheezing can create a feeling of helplessness. The anxiety patients feel during an asthma attack often stems from a deep-seated fear that their air supply might be cut off. *THE SINGLE BEST SOLUTION FOR REDUCING THE FEAR ASSOCIATED WITH ASTHMA IS TO BETTER UNDERSTAND YOUR PROBLEM SO THAT YOU KNOW JUST WHAT TO DO WHEN SYMPTOMS BEGIN . . . BEFORE THEY BEGIN.*

You must fully understand the program that has been outlined for you by your doctor, and know the name, dose, timing, and side effects of each medication. *BE SURE YOU KNOW WHICH MEDICATION TO TURN TO IF YOUR*

Why You Should Have a Written Summary of Your Asthma Medications

1. It makes it possible for your asthma to be treated promptly, without delay or confusion.

2. It reduces the uncertainty and panic often associated with a sudden asthma flare.

3. It specifies the proper dosage and timing of each of your medications, as well as the proper order in which to take them.

4. It emphasizes your medication's potential side effects so that you can be on the lookout for them.

5. It reminds you of medications which you should avoid (such as aspirin).

6. It specifies the exact point at which you should notify your doctor.

7. It is a first step toward self-management of your asthma, once your program has been worked out by your doctor.

Table 4–1

ASTHMA FLARES AND THE POINT AT WHICH YOU SHOULD NOTIFY YOUR DOCTOR. Each of these points should be written down as part of a medication program such as the ones to be outlined in the next chapter. This is an important step for all asthma patients, because there should be no question in your mind as to which medication to turn to on a daily or emergency basis. By being prepared in advance and knowing exactly what to do if your asthma flares, your anxiety about asthma will decrease (see Table 4–1).

A Home Peak-Flow Meter Will Measure Your Lung Function. Just as your doctor monitors your progress with a breathing test (spirometry), you can do the same with a peak-flow meter designed to measure your breathing capacity at home. You simply blow into the peak-flow meter and then compare the result with the normal predicted level and with your results from prior days. If your peak-flow level drops and you notice that your asthma symptoms seem worse, you should proceed with the steps outlined by your doctor for this situation in your management plan. You should notify your doctor early if your asthma is out of control and the back-up medications suggested in your management plan do not seem to be working.

Review the Factors That Trigger Your Asthma Symptoms and Work Out a Plan to Avoid Them or to Anticipate Them with Medications. If you are sensitive to environmental allergens, either at home or in the work place, efforts to limit your exposure or to pretreat yourself with medications prior to exposure can improve your breathing status. For example, precautions in the home to avoid dust exposure (especially in the bedroom) can markedly reduce asthma symptoms (see page 190). If you are sensitive to the seasonal pollens, simple measures such as using air conditioning and keeping the windows closed, especially in the early morning hours, can make a difference (see page 188).

If you find that your asthma symptoms are worse with exercise or with exposure to pets, review this with your doctor so that a preexercise or preexposure medication schedule can be worked out. For example, if your asthma symptoms become worse when you visit the home of a friend who has a pet, it may be possible to avert symptoms by using a bronchodilating inhaler prior to your visit. A bronchodilating inhaler can also block exercise-induced asthma (see page 158).

If you take asthma medications on a daily basis and you develop asthma symptoms from an upper respiratory infection, your management plan should indicate what to do. By knowing in advance the medications you will need, you can have these medications already on hand when the situation arises. Advance preparation is especially important for asthma patients in view of the fact that asthma flares tend to occur at night. If you notice that mucus from your nose or chest is green or yellow in color as opposed to being clear, you should contact your doctor, as an antibiotic may be necessary.

Asthma Patients Are Well Advised to Avoid Taking Aspirin, especially if your asthma symptoms flare when you take aspirin. If there is a specific reason for you to use aspirin, you should first discuss this with the doctor who manages your asthma. Asthma patients who are sensitive to aspirin should also avoid products that contain aspirin (such as Percodan, Midol, and Empirin) and products that cross-react with aspirin (such as Motrin, Advil, Naprosyn, and Indocin), and yellow food dye #5 (see Tables 2–3 and 2–4). Acetaminophen (such as Tylenol) should be used in place of aspirin by asthma patients sensitive to aspirin (see Table 2–5).

Sulfites which are added to various foods and medications, including some asthma medications (see page 47), can trigger asthma symptoms in certain individuals. If you notice that your asthma is worse when you are exposed to sulfites, be sure to discuss this with your doctor so that consideration can be given to ways in which you can avoid them.

Be Certain That Your Asthma Doctor Is Aware of Any Other Medical Problems You May Have and Any Medications Prescribed for You by Other Doctors. Your doctor needs to be familiar with your entire medical history. In particular, your doctor should be aware if you have a history of any heart, thyroid, liver, or blood pressure problems, as there may be a need to change the approach to your asthma care. For example, if you have a liver problem, this must be taken into consideration if you take theophylline for your asthma—since theophylline is broken down in the liver, your theophylline dose may have to be lower than it otherwise would be. If you have any heart problems, it is preferable for you to use an inhaled bronchodilator as opposed to an oral bronchodilator, as the inhaled medications tend to have less effect on the heart. Also, you should be sure to tell your asthma doctor if you have a hiatal hernia, since this condition can trigger asthma symptoms when stomach contents that are regurgitated up the esophagus (feeding tube) then pass into the airways (see Chapter 16).

Medications Called Beta Blockers, Which Are Used to Treat Heart Problems, Headaches, and Glaucoma, Must Be Avoided by All Asthma Sufferers. A group of medications called beta blockers are commonly used by cardiologists to slow the heart rate and thereby reduce the work of the heart. Since beta blockers can lead to a worsening of asthma symptoms, this group of medications should not be taken by asthma patients. Beta blockers are also found in eye drops for treatment of glaucoma and are often prescribed for difficult-to-manage headaches. The most commonly used beta blocker is propranolol (Inderal).

Sedatives Should Be Avoided When You Are Having Asthma Symptoms. When your asthma flares, you need to be as alert as possible so that you can breathe to the best of your ability. You may become fatigued during an asthma flare with the effort of breathing and have the desire to sleep, but your asthma symptoms will often prevent you from falling asleep. Although it might seem logical to take a sleeping pill, sedatives must never be used when you are having asthma symptoms. Sedatives should also not be given to "relax" the asthma sufferer in the hope that this will improve asthma symptoms. The danger with the use of sedatives during an asthma flare is that they tend to suppress the urge to breathe as well as to cough up accumulated secretions. This can lead to a drop in the blood's oxygen level and an increase in the blood's carbon dioxide level. If this condition progresses, the result could be the need to have your breathing supported with a breathing tube and mechanical ventilation.

Breathing Exercises Can Be Helpful When an Asthma Attack Begins. Breathing exercises provide a form of relaxation that can be of benefit to some patients during an asthma attack. However, it would be a mistake to rely on breathing exercises alone to control an asthma flare. Breathing exercises are meant to supplement, not to replace, the medications prescribed by your doctor. As always, if your asthma medications do not seem to be controlling your symptoms, you should contact your doctor early on. As long as this rule is not broken, breathing exercises are fine for those patients who find them of benefit. An outline of suggested breathing exercises is presented in Figure 4–1.

Smoking by Asthma Patients Is Unwise. Cigarette smoking poses the single greatest avoidable health risk today. The risk of lung cancer as well as the risk of irreversible lung damage such as emphysema are greatly increased in cigarette smokers. Smoking (either tobacco or marijuana) poses an additional risk for the person with asthma whose sensitive airways are easily irritated by smoke. Many patients experience asthma symptoms not just when they themselves smoke, but also when they are exposed to cigarette smoke from those around them. If this is the case for you, it is worth the effort to avoid smoke-filled rooms and to ask others not to smoke in your presence. If you smoke cigarettes and have thought about stopping or have tried unsuccessfully to stop, discuss this with your doctor as there are available a number of reliable, successful, and relatively inexpensive smoke cessation centers. Your local lung association is also a good source of information in this regard. Often, however, many people find that the only alternative is to stop "cold turkey."

If Your Asthma Symptoms Are Made Worse by Emotional Upset, Discuss This Openly with Your Doctor. Emotional upset cannot cause a person to have asthma, but it can cause asthma symptoms to flare or make asthma symptoms worse in a person who has the underlying problem of asthma (see page 247). If you feel that your emotional state contributes to your asthma symptoms, be sure to discuss this with your doctor. You should also tell your doctor if you tend to ignore your asthma or feel a sense of helplessness when asthma symptoms occur. The tendency to ignore asthma symptoms, hoping that they will go away, is a serious habit. If counseling by a psychiatrist or psychologist is suggested, view it as a positive suggestion that can help you help yourself.

Never Change Your Medication Program Without First Discussing It with Your Doctor. The purpose of a medication program is to outline exactly what you are to do

Breathing Exercises for Relaxation

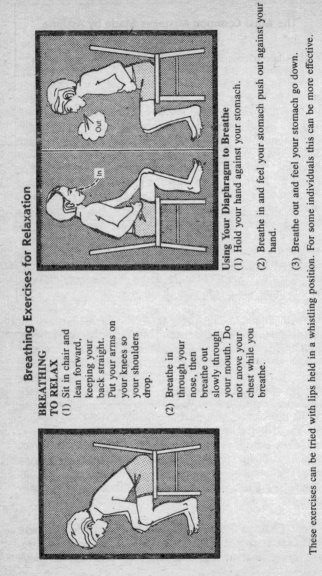

BREATHING TO RELAX

(1) Sit in chair and lean forward, keeping your back straight. Put your arms on your knees so your shoulders drop.

(2) Breathe in through your nose, then breathe out slowly through your mouth. Do not move your chest while you breathe.

Using Your Diaphragm to Breathe

(1) Hold your hand against your stomach.

(2) Breathe in and feel your stomach push out against your hand.

(3) Breathe out and feel your stomach go down.

These exercises can be tried with lips held in a whistling position. For some individuals this can be more effective.

Figure 4-1

The Most Common Mistakes Made by Asthma Patients

1. Failure to recognize the potential risks of overusing an asthma inhaler.

2. Delay in using asthma medications in the mistaken belief that asthma symptoms will subside on their own.

3. Assuming that because one pill helps to control asthma symptoms, two or more pills will work even better.

4. Allowing asthma symptoms to linger without notifying your doctor, so that a trip to the emergency room becomes unavoidable.

5. Refusing your doctor's recommendation to take steroids to treat an acute asthma flare, even though short-term steroid use carries little risk of steroid side effects and does not lead to steroid dependency.

6. Relying on your memory of your doctor's instructions rather than a written medication program.

Table 4–2

on a daily basis, in order to be as free as possible of asthma symptoms. If any of your medications are not providing relief or are not convenient to use or are causing unpleasant side effects, be sure to discuss this with your doctor so that your program can be amended. It must be emphasized that your medication program is an agreement between you and your doctor—the terms of the agreement can be changed whenever necessary, but the changes should be understood and agreed upon by both you and your doctor. To make changes on your own is not wise, as there may be very specific reasons why you are using a certain program. Be sure to avoid the mistakes often made by asthma patients listed in Table 4–2.

Never Change Your Theophylline or Steroid Dose Without Your Doctor's Approval. When not used properly, theophylline carries the potential for serious side effects.

As the dose of theophylline that is correct and safe for you has been carefully determined by your doctor, never increase or decrease that dose on your own. For example, it would be wrong to think that if you normally take one theophylline pill, two pills would work better during an asthma flare. In addition, never substitute a brand of theophylline or a generic theophylline product for the theophylline brand prescribed by your doctor without first consulting with him.

AS WITH ALL ASTHMA MEDICATIONS, STEROID DOSING SHOULD BE MANAGED BY YOUR DOCTOR, since there are potentially serious side effects with long-term steroid use. You should never take more steroids than your doctor prescribes, and you should also never alter your dosing schedule on your own. In addition, it can be dangerous to suddenly stop taking steroids even if you are feeling fine, since in some individuals this can cause asthma to flare. One of the goals of asthma management is to use as little steroid on a regular basis as possible. However, in trying to attain this goal, you must rely on your doctor's expertise.

Don't Get Caught in the Trap of Overusing Your Inhaler. Excessive use of your bronchodilating inhaler has the potential of causing irregular heartbeats. In addition, if you try to bring your asthma symptoms under control with the excessive use of an inhaler, this prevents you from notifying your doctor early enough when symptoms fail to respond, in the hope that the inhaler alone will be sufficient. The result of inhaler abuse more often than not is a trip to the doctor's office or hospital emergency room that often could have been prevented.

"Back-Up" Medications and When to Call Your Doctor. It is essential that your medication program be in writing. In addition to your routine medications, your medication program should also include back-up medications and practical suggestions for use when your routine medications fail to bring asthma symptoms under control. *BE CERTAIN THAT YOU HAVE DISCUSSED THESE BACK-UP PROVISIONS WITH YOUR DOCTOR IN ADVANCE, AND THAT*

THIS INFORMATION IS INCLUDED IN YOUR WRITTEN MEDICATION PROGRAM.

Some patients find a written medication program offensive as they believe that they can remember exactly what to do at each step. These are the patients that I worry about the most. They are more likely not to follow explicit instructions for the proper use of the prescribed medications, and to panic when asthma symptoms flare because they are unsure what to do. The effort involved in writing down and fully understanding the medications and suggestions of your doctor pays great dividends when asthma symptoms flare.

By following your routine medication program carefully, using your back-up plan when necessary, and calling your doctor early if the back-up plan proves unrewarding, the need for emergency hospital and doctor visits will be reduced. Even patients who rarely have symptoms benefit from having a clear-cut written medication program. The reason is that when asthma symptoms begin, there should not be any confusion about what to do. You should call your doctor if the back-up medications and suggestions fail to work, if you need reassurance or confirmation that you are following the correct steps, or if your asthma flare is severe or somewhat different than usual. By knowing what to do in advance, you will feel a sense of self-confidence which will reduce your anxiety whenever your asthma symptoms flare. Suggestions for appropriate steps to take when asthma symptoms flare are outlined in Table 4–3.

Steps to Take When Asthma Flares

1. Try to relax and stay calm.

2. Leave the area if there is an offending agent which is triggering your symptoms (such as a dog or cat, dust, cigarette smoke).

3. Refer to your medication program—use your first step medication (such as an inhaled or oral Adrenalin-like bronchodilator).

4. Drink plenty of clear liquids which are not too cold.

5. Perform your breathing exercises if they have been helpful in the past, or relax by watching television or listening to music.

6. Use your back-up medication (such as theophylline) if your first step medication proved unrewarding.

7. Notify your doctor if your medications fail to bring relief within the expected time period, or if your asthma symptoms are particularly severe, or if there is any sign of an infection requiring antibiotics.

Table 4–3.

◇ 5 ◇

The Asthma
Management Program

An asthma management program is an outline of the instructions and recommendations given by your doctor after he has reviewed your asthma history. A careful medical history with emphasis on the frequency, location, and timing, as well as the characteristics or severity of symptoms (see Table 5-1), is the key to planning an individualized asthma management program. When you see your doctor, it would be helpful for you to keep in mind the points summarized earlier in your asthma case history (page 9).

This chapter presents eleven sample management programs describing avoidance suggestions and medication choices for symptoms of varying severity. *THESE PROGRAMS ARE EXAMPLES AND SHOULD NOT BE USED INDEPENDENTLY OF YOUR DOCTOR'S EXPLICIT INSTRUCTIONS.* The sample program that most closely matches your symptoms can serve as a guide for a written asthma program prepared by you in accordance with your doctor's instructions. Be sure that your program includes the key points outlined in Table 5-2. You should ask your doctor to review your written medication program to ensure its accuracy and completeness.

A written asthma treatment plan is essential for successful self-management of your asthma (see Table 4-1, page 137). It will enhance your understanding and management of your

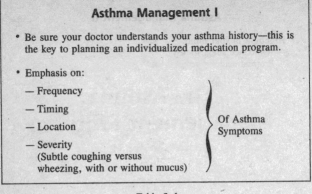

Table 5–1

asthma, and will also facilitate informed communication with your doctor. A comprehensive written management plan affords you the confidence that you will be prepared to deal effectively with your asthma episodes, thereby minimizing the panic and fear often associated with asthma attacks. By knowing the steps to take and the length of time for the appropriate medication to bring relief, you can frequently abort an asthma attack at the onset and avoid a trip to the hospital for emergency treatment. *YOUR MEDICATION PROGRAM SHOULD CLEARLY DELINEATE THE POINT AT WHICH SELF-MONITORING SHOULD BE STOPPED AND YOUR PHYSICIAN SHOULD BE CONTACTED.*

For Patients with Infrequent Asthma Symptoms— Sample Programs #1 through #3

Sample Program #1. This program is appropriate for a person with infrequent asthma symptoms. Once the patient's infrequent symptoms subside, he feels fine and his lung function returns to normal. Even the doctor cannot tell for sure that this patient has asthma on a "good" day. Yet this patient needs to know what to do if his asthma flares, even if asthma symptoms are infrequent. In addition, if exposure to a known allergen (such as cat or dog dander) causes asthma symptoms,

---

Asthma Management II

* Highlight in your mind:
  — Avoidance suggestions
  — Pretreatment suggestions

* Emphasize:
  — Proper techniques for medication use
  — Compliance with your medication program

* Be sure you understand:
  — Benefits and risks of each medication

* Don't neglect:
  — Prompt treatment of complicating situations (infections) as well as asthma flares
  — Being well-informed about your asthma
  — Your psychological status—panic and fear associated with asthma flares (if applicable)

Table 5–2

the patient should understand how to use preexposure measures to try to prevent symptoms from developing. In my experience, patient preparation and education have proven to be one of the most important ingredients to successful asthma management for all people who have asthma, even for those with infrequent symptoms.

Sample program #1 emphasizes the inhaled medication route as the first line of treatment. In addition to acting at the site of the problem (the airways), the inhaled route has the advantage of a rapid onset of action. Opening of the airways occurs within fifteen minutes. Use of the inhaler twenty minutes prior to exposure to a known allergen may block asthma symptoms from developing. Proper inhaler technique is important in order to achieve the greatest benefit from inhaled medications (see page 68). Patients often think that they use their inhalers properly when in fact they do not. Ask your doctor or his nurse to observe you while using an inhaler to be certain that your technique is proper. Newer inhalers which act more directly on the airways with less stimulation of the

Sample Program #1:
For Patients with Infrequent Asthma Symptoms
Who Do Not Use Asthma Medications Routinely

Begin this program at the onset of asthma symptoms:

- Use your **bronchodilating inhaler**, such as:
  - Albuterol (Proventil or Ventolin)

    or

  - Terbutaline (Brethaire)

    or

  - Metaproterenol (Alupent or Metaprel)

    — Dosage: 2 puffs spaced by 5 minutes—never to exceed 2 puffs every 4–6 hours. Do not overuse your inhaler.
    — Follow the instructions for inhaler use on page 68.
    — This medication begins to work rapidly (within minutes).
    — Side effects can include shakiness and jitteriness.
    — Can be used 20 minutes prior to exposure to a known allergen.

- Add your **back-up medication** if the inhaled medication alone is ineffective to relieve your symptoms:
  - A rapidly acting theophylline product (such as Slo-Phyllin or Elixophyllin tablets or liquid)

    — Dosage: _____ (# of) tablet(s) of _____ mg pills every 6 hours or _____ teaspoon(s) or tablespoon(s) every 6 hours.
    — This medication works within 2 hours and lasts 6 hours.
    — The most common side effects are nausea, vomiting, diarrhea, headaches, jitteriness, and restlessness.

- Contact your doctor promptly if your back-up medication fails to provide relief within _____ hour(s).

heart are preferable. This group includes inhalers such as albuterol (Ventolin or Proventil), terbutaline (Brethaire), and metaproterenol (Metaprel or Alupent). Inhalers containing isoproterenol (which is a greater stimulant of the heart than the newer inhalers) are still commonly prescribed but are less preferable for routine use. Over-the-counter inhalers (such as Primatene and Bronkaid) are best avoided.

You may experience shakiness or jitteriness with use of your inhaler. This is a normal reaction. However, if these side effects are excessive or if you notice palpitations in your chest, notify your doctor. Finally, it is important to note that for patients with heart problems, inhaled medications are usually preferable to oral medications, as medications that are inhaled act more directly on the airways with less effect on the heart than medications that are taken orally.

A back-up medication should be prescribed and kept on hand, to be used if the inhaled medication does not relieve asthma symptoms when used alone. Since in this situation your asthma symptoms are not responsive to your first-line medication, it is important to know in advance exactly what to do. Most often, the back-up medication is a short-acting theophylline product, which typically provides the greatest benefit within two hours. Examples of short-acting theophylline products are listed in Table 3–6. Once asthma symptoms are under control, a long-acting agent can be used for its greater convenience (lasting twelve hours, versus six hours for the short-acting theophylline products).

The long-acting medications such as Theo-dur and Slo-bid take far longer to become effective. For the patient's convenience, the doctor will sometimes instruct the patient to use long-acting theophylline in this setting, but to take it at eight-hour rather than twelve-hour intervals for the first day. This often eliminates the need to then switch from a short- to a long-acting theophylline product. However, if you find that there is a prolonged delay in relief when using long-acting theophylline as a back-up medication, discuss with your doctor the possibility of using a more rapidly acting theophylline product.

You need to know the typical side effects of theophylline, which include nausea, vomiting, diarrhea, headaches, jitteriness, and restlessness. If you experience any of these side effects, notify your doctor, as these symptoms may indicate that your dose of theophylline is too high.

If you have had to use your back-up medication and have noticed little relief, this is the time to notify your doctor if you have not already done so. It is important to emphasize that asthma is best managed early, to avoid the need for emergency hospital and doctor visits.

Sample Program #2. Program #2 is another alternative for patients with infrequent asthma symptoms. The program is ideally suited for younger children for whom mastering proper inhaler technique would be difficult or impossible. This program takes advantage of the products metaproterenol (Alupent or Metaprel) or albuterol (Ventolin or Proventil), which are liquid Adrenalin-like bronchodilators, to offer rapid relief of asthma symptoms until a theophylline product can take effect. Namely, both the metaproterenol or albuterol liquid and the theophylline are taken together at the first sign of asthma symptoms.

After the initial dose of each medication, the theophylline product is continued by itself in the prescribed dosage and at the appropriate time intervals, in order to provide sustained relief. The metaproterenol or albuterol is used again only as back-up if the theophylline by itself is ineffective in controlling asthma symptoms. Notify your doctor if this medication program proves unrewarding or if asthma symptoms are more severe than usual.

Potential side effects of each of the medications should be reviewed. Possible side effects of metaproterenol include jitteriness, nausea, and headache. The major side effects of theophylline include nausea, diarrhea, jitteriness, and headache. If you experience any of these side effects, you should review your medication program with your doctor.

The advantage of using a short-acting theophylline product in this program is to bring about rapid control of asthma symptoms. The disadvantage of short-acting theophylline is that it must be taken at six-hour intervals, which is not as convenient as taking long-acting theophylline every eight to twelve hours. This means that short-acting theophylline may not last through a typical night's sleep. Therefore, if asthma symptoms persist

Sample Program #2:
For Patients (Especially Children) with Infrequent Asthma Symptoms Who Do Not Use Asthma Medications Routinely

Begin this program at the onset of asthma symptoms:

- Metaproterenol in liquid or tablet form (Alupent or Metaprel)

  or

- Albuterol in liquid or tablet form (Ventolin or Proventil)

  and

- A rapidly acting theophylline liquid (such as Slo-Phyllin, Quibron, or Elixophyllin)

- Take both medications together for the first dose. Then take the theophylline alone every 6 hours.

- The metaproterenol or albuterol is used again only if the theophylline alone is ineffective.

Instructions:

- Metaproterenol or albuterol
  (a) _____ (# of) teaspoon(s) or _____ (# of) tablets at first sign of asthma symptoms, not to exceed one dose every 6–8 hours.

  (b) Oral metaproterenol and albuterol begin to work within 30–45 minutes, offering relief until the theophylline preparation begins to work.

  (c) Potential side effects include jitteriness, shakiness, restlessness ("hyped up" feeling), and nausea.

Instructions: (continued)

- Theophylline
  (a) _____ tablet(s) of _____ mg pills every 6 hours **or** _____ teaspoon(s) or tablespoon(s) every 6 hours.
       (# of)
  (b) _____ This medication works within 2 hours and lasts 6 hours.
  (c) The most common potential side effects are nausea, vomiting, diarrhea, headaches, jitteriness, and restlessness.
- Notify your doctor if this medication combination does not provide relief within 2 hours or if asthma symptoms are severe.

for several days, contact your doctor to ask if a long-acting theophylline product would be a worthwhile substitute.

Metaproterenol (Alupent or Metaprel) is approved for use
by children from ages six to twelve. On occasion, pediatri-
cians, pediatric allergists, or pulmonary specialists will use
metaproterenol in a child under the age of six. Needless to
say, in this circumstance careful adherence to the exact dosing
instructions, as well as close follow-up care with the child's
doctor, are essential. The newer Adrenalin-like oral bronchodilator albuterol (Ventolin or Proventil) recently has been
approved for use by children over two years of age. It is for
this reason that either metaproterenol or albuterol in liquid
form is the medication chosen for rapid relief of asthma
symptoms in this program. The pleasing taste of these liquids
is also an advantage for use by children.

Sample Program #3. Sample program #3 is similar to program #1 in that it is appropriate for adult asthma patients and
older children who have infrequent symptoms. This program
utilizes one of the newer oral Adrenalin-like medications as a
first-line product, such as albuterol or terbutaline, although metaproterenol is still acceptable. Terbutaline and albuterol are approved for use by adults and by children over age twelve. Since
it substitutes an oral medication for the inhaler used in program
#1, this program may be appropriate for individuals who have
strong aversions to using an inhaler, or who have such infrequent
asthma symptoms that they would not use an inhaler often
enough to master the proper technique. However, it should be
emphasized that the overall direction of asthma management
favors the use of inhaled rather than oral medications, because
they act more directly at the site of the problem (the airways),
with less effect on the rest of the body.

For patients with infrequent asthma symptoms, the oral
Adrenalin-like bronchodilator by itself is often sufficient.
Once an asthma flare begins to subside for these patients,
symptoms usually do not linger. If this is the case with your
asthma, be sure that your doctor is aware of this aspect of
your asthma history. Oral Adrenalin-like medications work
within thirty to forty-five minutes. This sample program also
provides a back-up theophylline medication, which you should

Sample Program #3:
For Patients with Infrequent Asthma Symptoms
Who Do Not Use Asthma Medications Routinely.

Begin this program at the onset of asthma symptoms:

- Use your oral Adrenalin-like bronchodilator such as:

  — Albuterol (Proventil or Ventolin)

  or

  — Terbutaline (Brethine or Bricanyl)

  or

  — Metaproterenol (Alupent or Metaprel)

  — Dosage: _____ (# of) tablet(s) of _____ mg pills, not to exceed 1 dose every 6–8 hours.

  — This medication begins to work within 30–45 minutes.

  — Side effects can include jitteriness, nausea, and headache.

- Add as **back-up medication** if the above medication is ineffective to relieve your symptoms:

  — A rapidly acting theophylline product (such as Slo-Phyllin or Elixophyllin tablets or liquid)

  OR

  — Dosage: _____ (# of) tablet(s) of _____ mg pills every 6 hours

  or _____ (# of) teaspoon(s) or tablespoon(s) every 6 hours.

  — This medication works within 2 hours and lasts 6 hours.

  — The most common side effects are nausea, vomiting, diarrhea, headaches, jitteriness, and restlessness.

• Contact your doctor promptly if your back-up medication fails to provide relief within _____ hour(s).

— A long-acting theophylline product (such as Slo-Phyllin Gyrocaps, Theo-dur, or Slo-bid)

— Dosage: _____(# of) pill(s) of _____(mg) mg tablet(s) or capsules, taken every 8 hours for the first 24 hours; then usually taken every 12 hours.

— This medication usually takes longer to start working than rapidly acting theophylline, but provides relief for a longer period of time.

— Potential side effects are the same as above for rapidly acting theophylline.

have on hand for use only if the Adrenalin-like product does not bring your symptoms under control.

For patients with infrequent asthma symptoms that are very mild, often a long-acting theophylline product can be used at eight-hour intervals for the first day, then tapered to the standard twelve-hour dosing schedule afterward. The use of a long-acting theophylline product in this fashion (instead of a short-acting theophylline product, which must be taken at six-hour intervals) is more convenient for the patient and allows an uninterrupted night of sleep. In addition, in order to reduce confusion it is preferable to have only one theophylline product in the medication plan.

For Patients with Exercise-Induced Asthma—Sample Program #4

Sample Program #4. Program #4 presents treatment alternatives for individuals who have asthma only when they exercise. Patients should not follow this program for routine asthma symptoms.

Exercise-induced asthma follows a pattern in which asthma symptoms occur during exercise that is strenuous, continuous, and sufficient to increase the heart rate to 80 percent of the predicted heart rate for the patient's age group. In a person who has exercise-induced asthma, symptoms usually develop after six to twelve minutes of exercise. Symptoms are typically at their worst five to ten minutes after exercise has stopped. Asthma is more likely to occur with long distance running as opposed to football, baseball, or tennis, where there are short bursts of physical activity interspersed with frequent stops.

The mechanism thought to explain exercise-induced asthma is that strenuous exercise necessitates breathing heavily through the mouth. This bypasses the nose, which normally serves to warm and humidify air that travels to the airways. With rapid mouth breathing, the air reaching the airways is cooler, dryer, and lacking in humidification, thereby triggering the asthma response. Swimming is thought to be the best exercise for asthma patients, as the air just above the water line is already humidified.

By understanding these basic points about exercise-induced asthma, management suggestions become clear. Exercise-induced asthma is best managed before exercise begins. One helpful technique is to use a warm-up period just prior to exercise, so that you can try to get through the critical first fifteen minutes of exercise without developing asthma symptoms. It is during this time period that exercise-induced asthma symptoms usually occur. Other techniques include using a face mask or scarf when exercising in cold weather to partially warm the air, and taking one of several acceptable medications to block asthma symptoms before they start. By following these basic suggestions, most asthma patients should be able to take part in exercise. Needless to say, the extent of exercise depends upon the person's overall health and physical condition.

Medication used to block exercise-induced asthma should be taken before exercise begins. The inhaled bronchodilators such as albuterol, terbutaline, or metaproterenol are clearly the preferred first step medications. They are best taken twenty minutes before exercise. Albuterol (Proventil or Ventolin), which has the advantage of working within minutes and lasting up to six hours, is presently considered the best medication choice to block exercise-induced asthma. As indicated in sample program #4, the albuterol dosage is two puffs of the inhaler spaced by five minutes. The ease of carrying and using the inhaler helps to minimize any self-consciousness a child might feel in this regard. School officials (such as the school nurse, physical education teachers, and coaches) should be aware that your child uses an asthma inhaler, so that this does not become an issue in front of the other children.

Interestingly, lung function actually improves during the first few minutes of exercise, thought to be as a result of the body releasing its own adrenalin in response to the physical exercise. This initial bronchodilation can be misleading, however, as asthma symptoms usually begin in susceptible individuals after several minutes of exercise. Some patients report that they are sometimes able to "run through" asthma symptoms during exercise simply by continuing to exercise without stopping. However, if you have exercise-induced asthma, you should discourage the temptation to skip your

Sample Program #4:
Preventative Treatments for Exercise-Induced Asthma

Choose only one of the following 4 options. Also see Table 2-2 for practical suggestions concerning exercise-induced asthma.

- *Option # 1*—A bronchodilating inhaler:
  - Albuterol (Proventil or Ventolin), **or**
  - Terbutaline (Brethaire), **or**
  - Metaproterenol (Alupent or Metaprel)

  Option # 1 is the most preferable of the 4 options.

  - 2 puffs (spaced by 5 minutes) taken 20 minutes before exercise, then 2 puffs every 4–6 hours if you begin to have asthma symptoms.

  - Potential side effects include shakiness and jitteriness.

- *Option # 2*
  - Cromolyn sodium (Intal)

  - 1 capsule via spinhaler or 2 puffs via inhaler 20 minutes before exercise.

  - A bronchodilating inhaler can be used prior to using cromolyn.

  - Is essentially free of side effects but should not be used if you are actively wheezing, as it can serve as an airway irritant.

- *Option # 3*—An oral Adrenalin-like bronchodilator:
  - Albuterol (Proventil or Ventolin), **or**
  - Terbutaline (Brethine or Bricanyl), **or**
  - Metaproterenol (Alupent or Metaprel)

  - ½–1 tablet taken orally ½ hour before exercise, then ½–1 tablet every 8 hours if you begin to have asthma symptoms.

  - Potential side effects include jitteriness, shakiness, restlessness, and nausea.

- *Option #4*
  - Theophylline: Take your routine dose so that it is timed to reach its peak when exercise begins.

  - The most common potential side effects are nausea, vomiting, diarrhea, headaches, jitteriness, and restlessness.

- Add as **back-up medication** if your preventative medication (outlined above) fails to block your asthma symptoms:
  - A rapidly acting theophylline product (such as Slo-Phyllin or Elixophyllin tablets or liquid)

  - Dosage: _____ (# of) tablet(s) of _____ mg pills every 6 hours
    or
    _____ (# of) teaspoon(s) or tablespoon(s) every 6 hours.
  - This medication works within 2 hours and lasts 6 hours.
  - Side effects can include nausea, vomiting, diarrhea, headaches, jitteriness, and restlessness.

- Contact your doctor promptly if your back-up medication fails to provide relief within _____ hour(s) preexercise medication in the hope that you won't need it, because the medication will not work to block an asthma flare once symptoms have begun. With the success of the currently available medications, it seems wise to pretreat yourself with the prescribed medication routinely before exercise if you have a pattern of developing asthma symptoms during exercise.

Alternatives to the inhaled bronchodilators include cromolyn sodium (Intal), oral Adrenalin-like bronchodilators, and theophylline. If an inhaled bronchodilator proves unrewarding, cromolyn sodium is an excellent alternative. Often the inhaled bronchodilator can be used prior to using cromolyn, to open the airways first and improve cromolyn's access to the airways. Cromolyn is best used twenty minutes before exercise. It blocks the exercise-induced asthma response for at least two hours. Cromolyn is also an excellent choice for children who are unable to use inhaled bronchodilators.

As outlined in program #4, another alternative to the medications discussed above for blocking exercise-induced asthma is the use of an oral Adrenalin-like bronchodilator. Medications such as albuterol (Proventil or Ventolin), terbutaline (Brethine or Bricanyl), or metaproterenol (Alupent or Metaprel) are all acceptable choices. Your doctor will prescribe the appropriate dose. The medication is best taken one hour before exercise to block the exercise-induced asthma response. The drawback of the oral Adrenalin-like medications is that they often stimulate the heart and sometimes cause shakiness. These side effects often pass with time or with a reduction of the dose. However, it is for these reasons that the inhaled method of administration is usually preferable.

Theophylline is another alternative for blocking exercise-induced asthma, if the proper dose is timed to reach its maximum effect at the usual time for exercise. As mentioned previously, a blood theophylline level of 10 to 20 micrograms per milliliter of blood serum is considered therapeutic, providing the greatest benefit with the least risk of side effects. It often takes several doses of theophylline to achieve this blood level. Therefore, relying on a single dose of theophylline to block exercise-induced asthma, although possible, is not ideal. For a patient who routinely takes theophylline, the medication schedule could be timed so that the theophylline reaches its peak at the usual time for exercise. For example, if long-acting theophylline is taken on a 10:00 A.M. and 10:00 P.M. schedule, the morning dose of theophylline should reach its maximum effect at approximately 4:00 P.M., a typical time for children to exercise after school. Your doctor can check the peak theophylline level (obtained six hours after the morning dose) to be certain that an adequate level of theophylline has been achieved. Often an additional medication such as an inhaled bronchodilator is needed during exercise along with theophylline. There is no contraindication to using a theophylline product as well as a bronchodilating inhaler at the same time, even during exercise.

An approach to exercise-induced asthma that is often overlooked is to be certain that the nose is as clear as possible. As discussed previously, the nose serves to humidify and warm the air going into the airways. When this does not take place, the cold dry air drawn directly into the airways can trigger asthma symptoms in someone who has asthma. If the nose is frequently stuffy (often as a result of allergies), the patient probably breathes through the mouth even during mild exercise, thus triggering asthma symptoms. Appropriate treatment of the nose can often help to reduce the need for mouth breathing during less strenuous exercise.

Although exercise-induced asthma usually subsides without treatment within one hour, you need to know what to do if symptoms continue or are troublesome. Suggestions for this are outlined in sample program #4. You should be sure that you are familiar with the steps your doctor recommends for you. One suggestion is to use your inhaler again by taking two additional puffs spaced by five minutes. If this proves unrewarding, you should start taking the theophylline product your doctor has prescribed in your medication program. If asthma symptoms still do not seem to be subsiding, notify your doctor.

For Patients with Daily Yet Mild Asthma Symptoms— Sample Programs #5 through #7

The programs that follow are for people who have asthma on a daily basis. These individuals often report symptoms ranging from a subtle yet persistent cough to intermittent wheezing during the day. These patients often require routine medication to bring their asthma symptoms under control.

Sample Program #5. This program is designed for patients who have mild asthma symptoms on a daily basis. A long-acting theophylline preparation is ideal for these patients, as it only has to be taken two or three times a day. This makes it much easier to remember to take the medication. In addition, when long-acting theophylline products (such as Theo-dur or Slo-bid) are taken on a routine basis, they tend to produce a constant theophylline level, which helps to avert symptoms throughout the day for most individuals. A single daily dose of a twenty-four-hour theophylline product (Theo-24 or Uniphyl) may be appropriate for some patients (see page 79). Young children can use a long-acting sprinkle theophylline preparation (see page 80). Reacquaint yourself with the potential side effects of theophylline, such as nausea, vomiting, diarrhea, or headache. Be sure to notify your doctor if you notice any of these symptoms.

Your blood theophylline level should be checked to be certain that your theophylline dose is not elevated above a safe level (20 milligrams per milliliter of blood serum). If your theophylline level is lower than the therapeutic range (namely, less than 10), there is no need to increase your theophylline dose if your asthma symptoms are well managed by your present dose. However, your breathing test (spirometry) should be rechecked by your doctor to confirm objectively your observation that your asthma is under control with your present theophylline dose.

If your theophylline level is low and you require medications in addition to theophylline to keep your asthma under control (especially steroids), your theophylline dose should be increased and monitored to bring your theophylline level into the therapeutic range. This will allow you to derive the greatest possible benefit from theophylline and possibly to reduce the need for additional medications that may carry greater chance of side effects.

Remember that there is no standard dose of theophylline correct for everyone. Your dose needs to be determined by

Sample Program #5:
For Patients with Daily yet Mild Asthma Symptoms

For routine use on a daily basis:	7:00 a.m.	10:00 a.m.	Noon	6:00 p.m.	10:00 p.m.
• **Long-acting theophylline** (such as Theo-dur or Slo-bid) _____ mg		✓			✓

— This is a timed medication, to be taken every 12 hours.
— Potential side effects include nausea, vomiting, diarrhea, headaches, jitteriness, and restlessness.
— Review the theophylline section, page 78.
— 24-hour theophylline (Theo-24 or Uniphyl) may be appropriate for some patients.
— Young children can use a long-acting sprinkle theophylline preparation (see page 80).

• If theophylline alone does not control your symptoms, add a **bronchodilating inhaler** such as: — Albuterol (Proventil or Ventolin) or — Terbutaline (Brethaire) or — Metaproterenol (Alupent or Metaprel)	— 2 puffs, spaced by 5 minutes, never to exceed 2 puffs every 4-6 hours. — Can be used routinely or only if needed. — Potential side effects include shakiness and jitteriness.

• Notify your doctor promptly if the addition of the bronchodilating inhaler fails to relieve your asthma symptoms, or if you experience any of the above-mentioned side effects.

your doctor on an individual basis, especially if you are not doing well.

For situations when long-acting theophylline by itself is insufficient to control your asthma, sample program #5 provides for the use of a bronchodilating inhaler such as albuterol or terbutaline. Be sure that you are using the inhaler properly in order to get the greatest possible benefit from the inhaled medication (see page 68). Be sure also to guard against overuse of your inhaler. If you notice that you are using your inhaler in excess of two puffs every four hours, you should notify your doctor immediately as reassessment of your program and additional medication may be necessary. Never delay contacting your doctor whenever your asthma symptoms are not controlled by the medications outlined in your program, taken in the proper amount and at the proper intervals.

Sample Program #6. Sample program #6 is similar to program #5 except that it relies on a bronchodilating inhaler as opposed to long-acting theophylline for routine use. The inhaled medication offers the advantage of acting directly to open the airways, with less effect on the rest of the body and consequently less potential risk of side effects than theophylline. Thus, this program may be a good starting point for patients who have routine asthma symptoms and are unable to tolerate theophylline, or who have heart or blood pressure problems. The bronchodilating inhaler, such as albuterol (Proventil or Ventolin), terbutaline (Brethaire), or metaproterenol (Alupent or Metaprel), is used every four to six hours.

You must have on hand a back-up theophylline product to turn to if your asthma symptoms flare. Use of the back-up theophylline should be sufficient to bring your asthma symptoms under control. Remember that if the theophylline product is not sufficient to control your symptoms, call your doctor for further suggestions.

Sample Program #7. This program utilizes cromolyn sodium (Intal) as the routine daily medication. A bronchodilating inhaler such as albuterol can be used first so that the cromolyn can better enter the airways. This program is often ideal for individuals who have routine asthma symptoms due

Sample Program #6:
For Patients with Daily yet Mild Asthma Symptoms

For routine use on a daily basis:	7:00 a.m.	Noon	6:00 p.m.	11:00 p.m.

• A bronchodilating inhaler such as:
— Albuterol (Proventil or Ventolin)
  or
— Terbutaline (Brethaire)
  or
— Metaproterenol (Alupent or Metaprel)
	✓	✓	✓	✓
				— 2 puffs, spaced by 5 minutes, never to exceed 2 puffs every 4–6 hours.
				— Potential side effects include shakiness and jitteriness.

• If your inhaler alone does not control your symptoms, add:
— A rapidly acting theophylline (Slo-Phyllin or Elixophyllin)
  or
	— Dosage: _____ (# of) tablet(s) of _____ mg pills every 6 hours
	  or
	  _____ (# of) teaspoon(s) or tablespoon(s) every 6 hours.
	— This medication works within 3 hours and lasts 6 hours.
	— The most common side effects are nausea, vomiting, diarrhea, headaches, jitteriness, and restlessness.			

• A long-acting theophylline (Theo-dur or Slo-bid)	— Dosage: _____ (# of) pill(s) of _____ mg tablet(s) or _____ mg capsule(s) taken every 8 hours: for the first 24 hours; then usually taken every 12 hours. — This medication usually takes longer to start working than rapidly acting theophylline, but provides relief for a longer period of time. — Potential side effects are the same as above for the rapidly acting theophylline.			
• Contact your doctor promptly if the addition of theophylline does not bring your symptoms under control.				

Sample Program #7:
For Patients with Daily Asthma Symptoms

	7:00 a.m.	Noon	6:00 p.m.	11:00 p.m.
For routine use on a daily basis:				
• Cromolyn sodium (Intal)	✓	✓	✓	✓

— A bronchodilating inhaler such as albuterol (Proventil, Ventolin), terbutaline (Brethaire), or metaproterenol (Alupent, Metaprel) can be used to open your airways prior to using cromolyn—2 puffs, spaced by 5 minutes.
— Cromolyn is inhaled through use of a spinhaler or an inhaler.
— Cromolyn is a preventative medication and therefore must be used routinely. It does not provide immediate relief during asthma symptoms.
— Potential side effects include irritation of the airways. Rinse your mouth and gargle after using cromolyn to remove any excess powder.

	7:00 a.m.	Noon	6:00 p.m.	11:00 p.m.
• If cromolyn is ineffective to prevent asthma symptoms, add as a back-up medication:				
— A rapidly acting theophylline (Slo-Phyllin or Elixophyllin)				
OR				
— A long-acting theophylline (Theo-dur or Slo-bid)				

— Dosage: _____ (# of) tablet(s) of _____ mg pills every 6 hours
   or
— _____ (# of) teaspoon(s) or tablespoon(s) every 6 hours.
— This medication works within 2 hours and last 6 hours.
— The most common side effects are nausea, vomiting, diarrhea, headaches, jitteriness, and restlessness.

— Dosage: _____ (# of) pill(s) of _____ mg tablet(s) or _____ mg capsule(s), taken every 8 hours for the first 24 hours; then usually taken every 12 hours.
— This medication usually takes longer to start working than rapidly acting theophylline, but provides relief for a longer period of time.
— Potential side effects are the same as above for the rapidly acting theophylline.

• Contact your doctor promptly if the addition of theophylline does not bring your symptoms under control.

to allergy. However, the use of cromolyn should not be restricted to these individuals. Cromolyn works by stabilizing the airways so that they are less reactive to irritants as well as to allergens. The key advantage of cromolyn is that it is essentially free of side effects. Therefore, a program relying on cromolyn is ideal for individuals who are unable to tolerate the potential side effects of theophylline or the Adrenalin-like bronchodilators. A back-up theophylline product or Adrenalin-like bronchodilator must be available in case asthma symptoms flare despite the cromolyn.

It is important for you to remember that cromolyn does not directly open the airways like theophylline or the bronchodilating inhalers. As a preventative medication, cromolyn does not provide any immediate improvement in asthma symptoms; rather, it provides a sustained effect of preventing asthma symptoms.

Cromolyn is inhaled either as a powder through the use of a spinhaler, as a mist produced from cromolyn's liquid form in a nebulizer, or through the use of a newly developed inhaler. Although the spinhaler may be somewhat inconvenient to carry about, the significant improvement in asthma symptoms noted by many patients who use cromolyn usually outweighs this minor inconvenience. Proper inhaler technique is essential for use of the spinhaler and the bronchodilating inhaler (see page 68). The frequency and timing of the cromolyn dose prescribed by your doctor should be written down, so that there is no uncertainty about the use of this medication.

On occasion, cromolyn can be irritating to the airways, causing minor short-lived asthma symptoms. However, if you notice asthma symptoms that are not transient, notify your doctor as soon as possible. Finally, it is best to gargle and rinse your mouth with warm water after using cromolyn, to remove any of the excess powder that might serve as an irritant to the throat.

For Difficult-to-Manage Asthma—Sample Programs #8 through #12

Sample programs #8 through #12 are more intensive programs, which utilize combinations of medications to control asthma symptoms. These programs are for individuals who have asthma that is more difficult to manage. You should review each of the medications in your program to be sure you understand their proper use. All asthma patients, and especially those with daily symptoms, should know the names and potential side effects of each of their prescribed medications. Since you take these medications on a routine basis, there probably will be situations in which you need to know specific information about your medications—for example, if you are out of town and run out of medicine, or if you need to seek emergency treatment.

Every medication in your program should be used in as ideal a manner as possible, in order to avoid the need for further medications such as steroids. If steroids are needed, they should also be used as ideally as possible (see page 110). If you are having difficulty with your asthma, notify your doctor *early*. It is a mistake to rely on a hospital emergency room to manage your asthma. By understanding the importance of being prepared for your asthma flares with a carefully designed medication program, you will need to turn to the emergency room less frequently, if at all.

Sample Program #8. Program #8 combines a long-acting theophylline product (such as Theo-dur or Slo-bid) with a bronchodilating inhaler, followed by a preventative inhaled product, in this case cromolyn sodium (Intal). An oral Adrenalin-like bronchodilator is available as a back-up medication. This program is designed for patients who have routine daily asthma symptoms and have not had good results with just theophylline and a bronchodilating inhaler. Since the potential next step is the use of steroids, attention to detail with each medication is vital.

Both your peak and your trough theophylline levels should be checked by your doctor. The peak level helps your doctor decide whether your theophylline dose is within your ideal range. A blood sample is taken when your theophylline dose is estimated to be at its peak; that is, at the approximate time when most of the theophylline should be in your bloodstream. For long-acting theophylline, this is usually around the sixth hour after the medication is taken.

To check your trough theophylline level, a blood sample is taken shortly before your dose of theophylline is normally taken. The trough level indicates whether the theophylline dose is sufficient to maintain a fairly constant level of theophylline from one dose to the next. If you notice that you are more likely to have asthma symptoms at the eighth to twelfth hour after taking long-acting theophylline, this could be a clue that your theophylline level is dropping off between doses. Often, moving the doses of theophylline closer (such as every eight hours for long-acting theophylline) can be quite helpful.

Never change your theophylline dose on your own without your doctor's approval. A serious mistake made by some asthma patients is to take several extra theophylline pills all at the same time when asthma starts to flare. This can sometimes lead to seizures and irregular heartbeats, which can be life threatening. You should rely on your doctor's instructions for the proper dose and dosing schedule of your theophylline.

Although some patients (especially children) find it mildly unpleasant to have a blood sample taken, blood theophylline levels can often provide the single most important piece of information to help your doctor manage your asthma without steroids.

In addition to theophylline, this program also includes a bronchodilating inhaler followed by inhaled cromolyn sodium (Intal). The bronchodilating inhaler is used to open the airways for the cromolyn sodium. Cromolyn is a preventative medication which helps to improve asthma symptoms over time when used on a routine daily basis. Cromolyn should not be used for immediate relief when asthma symptoms flare. Review sample program #7 above and Chapter 3 for further details concerning the use of cromolyn.

Proper inhaler technique is important. You should not simply assume that you use your inhaler properly. Rather, ask your doctor or his nurse to watch you use your inhaler. The inhaled medication should be used at six-hour intervals during the day. Proper spacing of the inhaled medication during the day can make a difference. Cromolyn sodium may be sufficient to block asthma symptoms and allow you to avoid steroids.

An oral Adrenalin-like bronchodilator such as albuterol or terbutaline tablets can be used if the preventative program outlined above proves unrewarding on its own. If the addition of

Sample Program #8:
For Patients with Asthma Which Is More Difficult to Manage

For routine use on a daily basis:	7:00 a.m.	10:00 a.m.	Noon	6:00 p.m.	10:00 p.m.	11:00 p.m.	
• Long-acting theophylline (such as Theo-dur or Slo-bid) _____ mg		✓		✓	✓		— This is a timed medication, to be taken every 12 hours. — 24-hour theophylline (Theo-24 or Uniphyl) may be appropriate for some patients. — Young children can use a long-acting sprinkle theophylline preparation (see page 80). — Potential side effects include nausea, vomiting, diarrhea, headaches, jitteriness, and restlessness. — Review the theophylline section, page 78.
• A bronchodilating inhaler such as: — Albuterol (Proventil or Ventolin) or — Terbutaline (Brethaire) or — Metaproterenol (Alupent or Metaprel), Followed by:	✓		✓	✓		✓	— 2 puffs, spaced by 5 minutes, never to exceed 2 puffs every 4–6 hours. — Potential side effects include shakiness and jitteriness.

	✓		✓		✓

- **Cromolyn sodium (Intal)**

  — Cromolyn is inhaled through use of a spinhaler or an inhaler.
  — Cromolyn is a preventative medication and therefore must be used routinely. It does not provide immediate relief during asthma symptoms.
  — Potential side effects include irritation of the airways. Rinse your mouth and gargle after using cromolyn to remove any excess powder.

- Add your **back-up medication** if the above program is ineffective to relieve your asthma symptoms:

- An oral Adrenalin-like bronchodilator such as:

  — Albuterol (Proventil or Ventolin)

  or

  — Terbutaline (Brethine or Bricanyl)

  or

  — Metaproterenol (Alupent or Metaprel)

  — $1/2$–1 tablet taken orally, then $1/2$–1 tablet every 8 hours if symptoms persist.
  — Potential side effects include jitteriness, shakiness, restlessness, and nausea.

- Contact your doctor promptly if your back-up medication fails to provide relief within _____ hour(s).

the oral bronchodilator is not sufficient to control your asthma symptoms, you should notify your doctor, as he may need to examine you or prescribe additional medications such as steroids. Also notify him about any signs of infection, as an antibiotic may be necessary as well. Clues that you might have an infection along with your asthma symptoms include fever or mucus from your nose or chest that is yellowish or greenish in color.

Sample Program #9. Sample program #9 is identical to program #8 except that an inhaled steroid preparation such as beclomethasone (Vanceril or Beclovent), triamcinolone (Azmacort), or flunisolide (AeroBid) replaces the cromolyn sodium. Inhaled steroids are an appropriate choice for patients who have routine daily asthma symptoms that have not been well managed with the use of theophylline and a bronchodilating inhaler. Patients who routinely have markedly increased mucus in their airways (one sign of airway inflammation) and whose routine spirometry is low despite the use of theophylline, often note improvement with the addition of inhaled steroids to their program.

As with cromolyn, the inhaled steroid serves as preventative medication and offers little immediate relief of asthma symptoms. The inhaled steroids improve asthma symptoms over time, so that episodes of asthma should become fewer and less severe. Inhaler technique for steroids is the same as for the inhaled bronchodilators. In this program, the inhaled bronchodilator is used first, to open the airways, followed by the inhaled steroid. Typical dosages range from two to four puffs of inhaled steroid taken four times a day. The risk of side effects is far less with inhaled steroids than with oral steroids. Some studies suggest that when inhaled steroids are used in conventional dosages, the risk of suppression of the adrenal gland is minimal.

This program also provides an oral bronchodilator (such as Ventolin, Proventil, Bricanyl, Brethine, Metaprel, or Alupent) for use as a back-up medication when the routine program outlined above fails to control asthma symptoms. Your doctor should be notified if your symptoms persist despite use of the back-up medication.

Sample Program #10. Program #10 expands upon program #9. The programs are identical except that in program #10 an oral Adrenalin-like bronchodilator is added for routine use. This program is appropriate for patients who frequently have daily asthma symptoms despite the use of inhaled steroids. These patients are often borderline candidates for routine oral steroid use. For some patients, the addition of the oral bronchodilator for routine use is sufficient to bring asthma symptoms under better control and possibly avert the need for oral steroids. Your breathing test should be carefully monitored to be certain that your breathing has in fact sufficiently improved with the addition of this medication.

Patients in this group often find a home nebulizer helpful during difficult times for administering a bronchodilating liquid such as metaproterenol or isoetharine. If the nebulizer is used, the patient then skips using his usual bronchodilating inhaler at that time. When symptoms are not acute, routine use of the nebulizer (in the morning, at 6:00 P.M., and/or at bedtime) can usually relieve asthma symptoms and not be overly inconvenient. Since the nebulizer is not easily portable, it is usually easier to rely on the bronchodilating inhaler for the noontime dose if you are not at home.

Sample Program #11. Program #11 is for patients who require oral steroids on a routine basis to keep their asthma under control. All medications short of oral steroids (such as a long-acting theophylline product and a bronchodilating inhaler, followed by a steroid inhaler) are still used. The oral steroids added to the patient's program are used in the lowest dosage range necessary to control asthma symptoms. Although oral steroids have been added, the other medications are still continued to keep the airways open and keep the dose of steroid to a minimum.

Oral steroids are the last medication that should be added to a routine asthma medication program. They are used in the lowest possible dosage when used on a routine basis. The need for oral steroids must be frequently reevaluated by your doctor. Oral steroids are best taken early in the morning, to reduce the risk of adrenal gland suppression and steroid side effects. Whenever possible, it is preferable to take oral steroids on an alternate day

Sample Program #9:
For Patients with Asthma Which Is More Difficult to Manage

For routine use on a daily basis:	7:00 a.m.	10:00 a.m.	Noon	6:00 p.m.	10:00 p.m.	11:00 p.m.	
• Long-acting theophylline (such as Theo-dur or Slo-bid) _____ mg and		✓			✓		— This is a timed medication, to be taken every 12 hours. — 24-hour theophylline (Theo-24 or Uniphyl) may be appropriate for some patients. — Young children can use a long-acting sprinkle theophylline preparation (see page 80). — Potential side effects include nausea, vomiting, diarrhea, headaches, jitteriness, and restlessness. — Review the theophylline section, page 78.
• A bronchodilating inhaler such as: — Albuterol (Proventil or Ventolin) or — Terbutaline (Brethaire) or — Metaproterenol (Alupent or Metaprel), Followed by:	✓		✓	✓		✓	— 2 puffs, spaced by 5 minutes, never to exceed 2 puffs every 4–6 hours. — Potential side effects include shakiness and jitteriness.

	✓	✓	✓	✓			✓
• An inhaled steroid product such as: — Beclomethasone (Vanceril) or — Triamcinolone (Azmacort) or — Flunisolide (AeroBid)						— Inhaled steroid is a preventative medication and therefore must be used routinely. It does not provide immediate relief during asthma symptoms. — The risk of side effects is far less with inhaled steroid than with oral steroid. — Potential side effects include irritation of the throat, and a condition called thrush. Rinse your mouth and gargle after using inhaled steroids to remove any excess medication. — Flunisolide (AeroBid) is usually used only twice a day.		

• Add your **back-up medication** to the above program if your asthma symptoms flare:

• An oral Adrenalin-like bronchodilator such as: — Albuterol (Proventil or Ventolin) or — Terbutaline (Brethine or Bricanyl) or — Metaproterenol (Alupent or Metaprel)	— ½–1 tablet taken orally, then ½–1 tablet every 8 hours if symptoms persist. — Potential side effects include jitteriness, shakiness, restlessness, and nausea.

• Contact your doctor promptly if your back-up medication fails to provide relief within _____ hour(s).

Sample Program #10:
For Patients with Asthma Which Is More Difficult to Manage

For routine use on a daily basis:	7:00 a.m.	10:00 a.m.	Noon	3:00 p.m.	6:00 p.m.	10:00 p.m.	11:00 p.m.	
• Long-acting theophylline (such as Theo-dur or Slo-bid) ____ mg and		✓				✓		— This is a timed medication, to be taken every 12 hours. — 24-hour theophylline (Theo-24 or Uniphyl) may be appropriate for some patients. — Young children can use a long-acting sprinkle theophylline preparation (see page 80). — Potential side effects include nausea, vomiting, diarrhea, headaches, jitteriness, and restlessness. — Review the theophylline section, page 78.
• A bronchodilating inhaler such as: — Albuterol (Proventil or Ventolin) or — Terbutaline (Brethaire) or — Metaproterenol (Alupent or Metaprel), Followed by:	✓		✓		✓		✓	— 2 puffs, spaced by 5 minutes, never to exceed 2 puffs every 4–6 hours. — Potential side effects include shakiness and jitteriness. — A home nebulizer can replace the inhaler during difficult asthma symptoms, using bronchodilating liquids such as metaproterenol (Alupent or Metaprel) or isoetharine (Bronkosol). Dosage: ____ cc of medication in ____ cc of saline.

- An inhaled steroid product such as:
  — Beclomethasone (Vanceril)
  or
  — Triamcinolone (Azmacort)
  or
  — Flunisolide (AeroBid)
  and

  — Inhaled steroid is a preventative medication and therefore must be used routinely. It does not provide immediate relief during asthma symptoms.
  — The risk of side effects is far less with inhaled steroid than with oral steroid.
  — Potential side effects include irritation of the throat, and a condition called thrush. Rinse your mouth and gargle after using inhaled steroids to remove any excess medication.
  — Flunisolide (AeroBid) is usually used only twice a day.

- An oral Adrenalin-like bronchodilator such as:
  — Albuterol (Proventil or Ventolin)
  or
  — Terbutaline (Brethine or Bricanyl)
  or
  — Metaproterenol (Alupent or Metaprel)

  — ½–1 tablet taken orally.
  — Potential side effects include jitteriness, shakiness, restlessness, and nausea.

- Contact your doctor promptly if this program does not control your asthma symptoms, as oral steroids may be necessary.

Sample Program #11:
For Patients with Asthma Which Is More Difficult to Manage

For routine use on a daily basis:	7:00 a.m.	10:00 a.m.	Noon	6:00 p.m.	10:00 p.m.	11:00 p.m.
• Long-acting theophylline (such as Theo-dur or Slo-bid) ____ mg and		✓			✓	

— This is a timed medication, to be taken every 12 hours.
— 24-hour theophylline (Theo-24 or Uniphyl) may be appropriate for some patients.
— Young children can use a long-acting sprinkle theophylline preparation (see page 80).
— Potential side effects include nausea, vomiting, diarrhea, headaches, jitteriness, and restlessness.
— Review the theophylline section, page 78.   ✓

	7:00 a.m.	10:00 a.m.	Noon	6:00 p.m.	10:00 p.m.	11:00 p.m.
• A bronchodilating inhaler such as: — Albuterol (Proventil or Ventolin) or — Terbutaline (Brethaire) or — Metaproterenol (Alupent or Metaprel), Followed by:	✓	✓	✓	✓		

— 2 puffs, spaced by 5 minutes, never to exceed 2 puffs every 4-6 hours.
— Potential side effects include shakiness and jitteriness.
— A home nebulizer can replace the inhaler during difficult asthma symptoms, using bronchodilating liquids such as metaproterenol (Alupent or Metaprel) or isoetharine (Bronkosol). Dosage: ____ cc of medication in ____ cc of saline.

	✓	✓	✓	✓	✓
• An inhaled steroid product such as: — Beclomethasone (Vanceril) or — Triamcinolone (Azmacort) or — Flunisolide (AeroBid) **and**					— Inhaled steroid is a preventative medication and therefore must be used routinely. It does not provide immediate relief during asthma symptoms. — The risk of side effects is far less with inhaled steroid than with oral steroid. — Potential side effects include irritation of the throat, and a condition called thrush. Rinse your mouth and gargle after using inhaled steroids to remove any excess medication. — Flunisolide (AeroBid) is usually used only twice a day.
• Oral steroids such as: — Prednisone or — Prednisolone or — Methylprednisolone (Medrol)					— _____ mg, taken at the specific time(s) prescribed by your doctor. — Oral steroids are best taken in the early morning and, if possible, every other day. — Oral steroids are best taken with food. — Never change your steroid dose or timing without your doctor's knowledge. — Review the potential steroid side effects. See Table 3–15, page 109. — If your asthma symptoms flare, a steroid boost may be necessary. This can only be done under your doctor's supervision.

- Add as **back-up medication** if the above program is ineffective to relieve your asthma symptoms:

  - An oral Adrenalin-like bronchodilator such as:
    - Albuterol (Proventil or Ventolin), or
    - Terbutaline (Brethaire or Bricanyl), or
    - Metaproterenol (Alupent or Metaprel)

    - ½–1 tablet taken orally, then ½–1 tablet every 8 hours if symptoms persist.
    - Potential side effects include jitteriness, shakiness, restlessness, and nausea.

- Contact your doctor promptly if your back-up medication fails to provide relief within _____ hour(s).

dosage schedule, since the risk of side effects is significantly less with alternate day steroids. The least desirable way of taking oral steroids is on a split daily schedule, with steroids taken both in the morning and in the evening (see page 110, Chapter 3 for a more complete discussion).

You should review the potential steroid side effects (Chapter 19). Any questions you have should be reviewed with your doctor. You should feel comfortable with the decision that steroids are necessary to control your asthma. If you do not feel comfortable, you should review your concerns with your doctor. While taking long-term oral steroids, an eye examination and a tuberculin skin test should be performed periodically. Careful periodic reevaluation of your need for steroids is also important.

If your asthma symptoms flare, a steroid ''boost'' may be necessary. Your doctor may direct you to take 30 to 40 milligrams of oral steroids as a onetime dose. The steroids are then gradually tapered down over several days to your routine dose. Oral steroids are best taken with food, as they can irritate the stomach. You should review the section on oral steroids for other suggestions in this regard (page 105).

If you require oral steroids on a daily basis and the dose is quite high (greater than 30 milligrams), consideration can be given to the use of steroid-reducing agents such as troleandomycin (see page 131). The addition to your program of a medication such as TaO should be closely supervised by your doctor.

Sample Programs #12 and #13—Creating Your Own Asthma Medication Program. Sample program #12 provides a general format for treatment appropriate for someone with infrequent asthma symptoms. Sample program #13 is a general format for a patient who requires routine asthma medication. Review the instructions that your doctor has given you and use these samples as a guide to organize your own asthma management plan for the medications prescribed by your doctor. You should review your outline with your doctor to be sure that it is accurate.

Sample Program #12:
Creating Your Own Asthma Medication Program:
If You Have Infrequent Asthma Symptoms and Do Not Require Asthma Medications Routinely
(Using your doctor's instructions)

Begin this program at the onset of asthma symptoms:

- (Medication prescribed by your doctor) — Dosage, instructions, side effects.

- Add your back-up medication if the above medication alone is ineffective to relieve your symptoms:
  - (Medication prescribed by your doctor) — Dosage, instructions, side effects.
    — Know when to contact your doctor.

- Special general measures of which to be aware (some examples):
  - Avoidance techniques.
  - Aspirin-containing products, medications which cross-react with aspirin.
  - Pretreatment for exercise-induced asthma.

- Review your written medication program with your doctor.

Sample Program #13:
Creating Your Own Asthma Medication Program:
If Your Asthma Symptoms Require Routine Medication
(Using your doctor's instructions)

For routine use on a daily basis:	7:00 a.m.	10:00 a.m.	Noon	3:00 p.m.	6:00 p.m.	10:00 p.m.	11:00 p.m.

- (Medication prescribed by your doctor)
  ___ mg

  (Check the times specified by your doctor.)
  — Instructions, side effects.

- (Any additional medications)

- Add a **back-up medication** to the above program if your asthma symptoms flare:

  — (Medication prescribed by your doctor)

  — Dosage, instructions, side effects.
  — Know when to contact your doctor.

- Special general measures of which to be aware (some examples):
  — Avoidance techniques.
  — Aspirin-containing products, medications which cross-react with aspirin.
  — Pretreatment for exercise-induced asthma.

- Review your written medication program with your doctor.

◇ 6 ◇

Environmental Influences

It is essential for the asthma patient to understand that his airways are supersensitive. As previously discussed, irritants such as cigarette smoke, perfumes, and newsprint can trigger asthma symptoms even if one is not allergic. Asthma symptoms can also be triggered in allergic asthma patients by various airborne allergens. Although the reasons are not fully understood, weather conditions (including temperature, humidity, and barometric changes) no doubt have impact on asthma as well. This section will review some of the many factors that can influence asthma symptoms and offer some practical suggestions and environmental precautions that have been shown to improve asthma symptoms.

General Principles. To determine which factors trigger your asthma symptoms (page 17), you must be a keen observer. If you notice that you begin to cough or wheeze when you are in a damp basement or in a dusty room, avoidance measures regarding molds or dust can improve your asthma symptoms. If you wake up early in the morning with asthma symptoms, consider that these symptoms may be due to your feather pillow or to a pet that is allowed in the bedroom. If you suffer from asthma symptoms in your home but are fine when you are traveling to another city, this should be brought to your doctor's attention. If you are fine on the weekend but troubled with asthma symptoms during the week, this distinction can help you to determine whether your asthma is made worse by an occupational irritant or cigarette smoke at work. Clearly, steps to improve your environmental exposures can improve your asthma symptoms, but the factors important to triggering your asthma must first be understood.

The Importance of a Diary. When asthma symptoms occur immediately after exposure to an airborne allergen or irritant, it is somewhat easier to correlate the exposure to the symptoms. When asthma symptoms occur on a delayed basis, often several hours after exposure (as can occur with several occupational exposures), it is much more difficult to identify what has triggered the asthma symptoms. It can be helpful to keep a diary of your day-to-day activities and the status of your asthma, and to review it periodically with your doctor, especially if your asthma is difficult to manage.

Overview of the Potential Factors. Factors that can influence asthma symptoms include allergens, irritants, and weather and climate changes. Allergens affect only patients who are allergic, while irritants and weather changes can affect all asthma patients. Yet nonallergic asthma patients can still find that their asthma is affected by allergens such as dust when these allergens act as irritants to trigger asthma symptoms.

Airborne Allergens. Allergens are capable of producing asthma symptoms in individuals who are allergic to the particular allergen and who have asthma. The allergens that cause asthma symptoms typically become airborne, directly striking the nose, eyes, or airways. As previously described (Figure 2–1, page 17), asthma symptoms can occur when the allergen comes in contact with the specific IgE antibody for that allergen sitting on the mast cells in the airways. The airborne allergens most commonly associated with asthma symptoms are pollens, house dust, mold spores, and animal danders. A brief review of each of these airborne allergens will now be presented.

Pollens. Pollen grains are the male counterpart in the reproductive cycle of seed-producing plants such as trees, grasses, ragweed, and flowering plants. Pollen grains are microscopic in size and light enough to be carried either by the wind or by insects. Lightweight, airborne pollen grains are the most frequent cause of allergic symptoms. Grass and ragweed pollens, for example, are light enough to be carried for miles by air currents. On the other hand, the pollens of brightly colored flowers such as roses or the goldenrod weed are heavier, and are usually carried by insects. Often travelers along highways spot the large gold-colored puffs of goldenrod and mistake it for ragweed. However, the pollen from goldenrod is too heavy to become airborne and therefore causes few asthma symptoms unless you actually are close enough to smell it.

Seasonal Pattern for Your Area. It is essential for you to know the seasonal occurrence for each of the allergens in your area of the country. Your local chapter of the Asthma and Allergy Foundation of America can provide this information. Appendix A offers a guide to the various regions of the country (see page 341). For example, in the northeastern and mid-Atlantic states, trees pollinate in the early spring while grasses pollinate in late spring and early summer. Pollen from the English plantain weed is often airborne at the same time as grass pollen. At times, a patient who has symptoms during the grass season is not truly grass allergic but sensitive to this weed instead. This distinction is well known to allergists. In the eastern and midwestern states, ragweed typically occurs in the later part of the summer and early fall (beginning around August 15), and persists until the first frost.

Pollen Counts. Pollen counts measure the amount of airborne pollen in the specific locale which is sampled. The specific number is often not as important as knowing that the pollen to which you are sensitive is now elevated. Pollen counts tend to be elevated when it is windy and dry. Rainfall and low temperatures generally lower the pollen count.

Avoidance Measures. The seasonal pollens are often quite difficult to avoid. Practical suggestions in this regard include:

(a) Keep your bedroom windows closed and use air conditioning as much as possible during the pollen seasons—as ragweed pollinates during the early morning hours, it is likely that your asthma will flare if you leave your bedroom window open. (b) If you use a window air conditioner rather than central air conditioning, be sure that it is set on the "circulate" mode rather than the "ventilate" mode, which takes in fresh air from the outside. (c) Use the air conditioner in your car, especially when driving on the highway. (d) Remember that weather conditions favoring the spread of pollen are dry, windy days. (e) Remember that ragweed tends to flourish in areas where the soil has been disturbed, such as along highways or at construction sites. (f) Consider using pretreatment medication regimens in anticipation of asthma symptoms if you can foresee unavoidable exposure to airborne pollens.

House Dust. As the airways of a person with asthma are supersensitive and ready to constrict in response to various stimuli, it is no wonder that various forms of dust can serve as irritants as well as allergens. As mentioned previously, an allergen (as opposed to an irritant) can cause the immune system of an allergic individual to form an IgE antibody specific to that allergen. The antibody develops with repeated exposure to the allergen over time, and sits on the mast cells in the patient's airways, ready to respond to the allergen on subsequent exposure. With reexposure, the mast cell releases chemical mediators (such as histamine) which can trigger asthma symptoms. Irritants, on the other hand, do not have IgE antibodies directed to them. Rather, they can directly trigger the airways to constrict.

Dust is derived from both living (organic) and nonliving (inorganic) sources. House dust is a mixture of various plant and animal (organic) as well as environmental (inorganic) substances. House dust contains insect debris, animal dander, human skin fragments, and food remnants, as well as bacteria and fungi. Another component of house dust is house-dust mites, microscopic insects that thrive on food debris and scales shed by human skin. House-dust mites can trigger allergic symptoms in both the nose and the chest. Once house dust is airborne, it can act both as an allergen (in patients who have an allergic tendency) and as an irritant. Dust from nonliving (inorganic) matter, such as dust from plasterboard or from roadways, acts as an irritant, not an allergen, to the airways of individuals who are sensitive to it.

Although it is nearly impossible to avoid dust completely, it is worthwhile for the person with asthma to try to reduce his exposure to it as much as possible. Allergists highlight the importance of reducing dust in the bedroom, since about one third of the day is usually spent there sleeping. Among asthma patients who followed dust precautions in these studies, asthma symptoms and the need for supplemental medications such as steroids were reduced significantly. Making the bedroom as dust-free as possible is the first step in dust control. Suggestions in this regard include:

1. Avoid clutter in the bedroom. Ornate furnishings and knickknacks are dust collectors. A minimal amount of furniture should be used. Wall decorations (such as pictures and pennants) and fabric-covered walls all collect dust. Washable curtains should be used instead of venetian blinds or heavy draperies. There should be no bookshelves in the bedroom.

2. The bedroom closet should be thoroughly cleaned and used only for the current season's clothing. There should be minimal storage in the bedroom closet. All clothing should be kept in place, and not left lying around. The door to the closet should be kept closed when the closet is not being used.

3. Hardwood or linoleum floors are preferable to carpeting. Frequent cleaning of floors (at least weekly) is recommended. Most patients prefer to have carpeting in the bedroom, although this requires greater effort in reducing dust. If carpeting is used, a tightly woven rug (especially one that is washable) is less likely to collect dust than is a shag carpet. Frequent and thorough vacuuming is essential.

4. Mattresses and box springs should be completely covered with allergen-proof casing. Zippers should be sealed with

tape. Be certain that you clean under the bed with your routine cleaning of the bedroom. There should be no storage under the bed.

5. Pillows should also be encased in allergen-proof casings. The pillow itself should be replaced every year or two. Hypoallergenic polyester materials such as Dacron are the best choice for pillows. Feather, kapok, and foam pillows should be avoided. Foam pillows can be a potential source of mold growth if perspiration gets into the foam.

6. Blankets, bedspreads, and mattress pads should all be washable. Sheets and other bedding are best washed in hot water. A bedspread should be kept on the bed during the day in order to collect dust. Both the blankets and pillows should be covered by the bedspread. The bedspread should be removed from the bed at night. Do not sleep with the bedspread. Quilts that serve as both the blanket and bedspread should not be used.

7. A child with asthma should be allowed to sleep with only one nonallergic stuffed toy, which should be frequently washed. There should be no other stuffed toys allowed in the bedroom.

8. Forced-air heating vents should be closed and sealed, unless there is a dust-filtering system or an electrostatic air cleaner on the central heating system. A piece of clean, damp cheesecloth can be placed over the vent to check to see if the filtering system is adequate, and will itself serve as a filtering system.

9. The bedroom should be thoroughly cleaned twice a week. Ideally, the allergic individual should not do the cleaning. However, if there is no alternative, a dust mask may be helpful. Dusting should be performed using a damp cloth, which will collect the dust, not just move it around. The asthma patient should stay out of the bedroom for several hours after a cleaning, as the dust is more likely to be airborne at that time.

10. Once the above steps have been taken, the bedroom then becomes a good place for the allergic child to play and study. Toys should be returned to another room for storage when the child is not playing with them in the bedroom.

11. Pets should never be allowed in the bedroom. Keep the bedroom door closed during the day to prevent the pet from entering the bedroom when you are away. It can take weeks of vacuuming to remove animal dander from the carpet and furniture.

Although these suggestions can seem overwhelming at first glance and patients often question whether they will make a difference, steps to reduce dust exposure can reduce asthma symptoms and possibly reduce the amount of medication necessary to control asthma symptoms. It is important to make the bedroom the asthma sufferer's haven. Finally, after all the work of putting the bedroom in order, be sure not to allow cigarette smoking there.

Molds. Molds (also referred to as mildew) can be found throughout the house, outdoors, and in certain foods. Molds produce lightweight spores as part of their reproductive process. It is these spores, spread by air currents, that can be associated with allergic symptoms, including asthma.

Although some molds do have seasons when they tend to flourish, mold spores are present in our environment both outdoors and indoors on a year-round basis. Molds tend to flourish when there is moisture and high humidity.

Common locations for mold growth and some practical suggestions for mold control are listed below:

1. Bathrooms are popular havens for molds. Be certain that your bathrooms are cleaned thoroughly, using a fungicide if necessary. Often proper ventilation of the bathroom can be sufficient to control mold growth. Shower curtains, bathroom tiles, and areas around plumbing fixtures (such as under the sink and behind the toilet) are usually the problem areas.

2. Damp basements provide ideal conditions for mold growth. Often the use of a dehumidifier is sufficient to control the situation. It is best to try to repair a leaky basement that becomes wet whenever it rains, as this situation constantly invites mold growth.

3. Humidifiers, vaporizers (including cold-mist vaporizers), and air conditioners are potential sources for mold growth. Spray-type humidifiers are preferable to drum-type, as water does not pool in them. If room vaporizers are used, the water should be changed daily and the base cleaned routinely.

4. Old pillows (especially foam pillows) and old mattresses can be sites for mold growth. As we perspire somewhat when we sleep, the moisture from perspiration can get into the pillow, thereby providing the conditions for mold growth. Change pillows frequently, typically every year or two.

5. Dried flowers and plants often contain molds. Dead leaves and plant debris should not be allowed to remain in potted plants. Mold growth can also occur within the soil. If you are considering repotting a plant, do it out of the house so as not to disperse mold spores inside. Remove plants and dried flowers from the bedroom.

6. Outdoor locations for mold growth include leaves, mulch, and compost piles as well as soil. Cutting the lawn, which liberates mold spores into the air, can lead to symptoms in mold-sensitive individuals. Mold growth is very dependent on the weather, favoring warm, moist conditions.

7. Some asthma patients report that some of the mold-containing foods—such as alcoholic beverages (beer and wines), aged cheeses, and vinegar—tend to cause subtle asthma symptoms. If you have noticed this, discuss it with your doctor. A more complete list of the mold-containing foods is presented in Table 2–7.

◇ 7 ◇

Allergy Immunotherapy
(Shots)

Allergy shots are small doses of the specific allergen to which you are allergic, and are given to reduce your sensitivity to the allergen. Allergy shots do take time to work (up to one to two years), but, if successful, they can reduce your need for medication and reduce your symptoms.

How Do Shots Work? Although a full explanation of how allergy shots work is not available, it is clear that they stimulate the body to produce an antibody of a different shape from that of IgE, called IgG. Because the structure of IgG is different, it cannot join to the mast cell and cause the release of histamine. Rather, IgG "blocks" the allergen from joining to the IgE antibody on the mast cell and thereby reduces your sensitivity. As the allergy shots are increased in strength over a period of time, the IgG antibody increases while the IgE antibody decreases. Although improvement is often noted between the first and second year of allergy shots, the shot program should be continued for three to five years at high dosage in order to achieve results of a more permanent nature.

Candidates for Allergy Shots. Allergy shots are usually reserved for individuals who are unable to avoid the offending allergen, who have allergy seasons that are longer in duration than a few weeks, and who have difficult symptoms that cannot be managed satisfactorily with medications alone. Assuming that the patient's history and skin test results indicate that allergy plays a role in asthma symptoms, asthma patients who are candidates for allergy shots include those who: (a) have difficult-to-manage asthma symptoms that have not been well controlled with medication alone; (b) have multiple allergies that result in year-round symptoms, necessitating daily medications; and (c) have asthma symptoms that have been more difficult during the pollen seasons, since the success with allergy shots is greatest with the seasonal pollens. Allergy shots can also be considered for individuals who are intolerant of the side effects of the available allergy medications and whose history and skin tests suggest that there will be a reasonable chance of success with the shots.

Accurate Diagnostic Procedures Are Essential. It is important that your allergic history and skin test results can be correlated accurately. For example, if you have asthma flares in the latter part of the summer and early fall and live in the northeastern United States, your allergist will check whether your allergy skin testing corresponds to the seasonal pattern for that area, with positive test results to ragweed, other weeds, or molds. Sensitivity to dust, molds, animal danders, and feathers are the usual allergens that explain year-round symptoms. As success with allergy shots do vary depending on your specific allergic sensitivity, it is essential that the decision of whether to begin a program of allergy shots be made with accurate information.

Success Rate with Allergy Shots. Although only a few studies clearly show that allergy shots reduce the incidence of asthma symptoms, allergists for years have observed this to be the case. Studies are clear-cut in showing that allergy shots do reduce the extent of symptoms and the need for medications in allergic rhinitis (hay fever). More studies are presently under way to evaluate the success of allergy shots for asthma. For example, studies concerning asthma due to allergy to cats have shown that allergy shots can be helpful in improving asthma symptoms. In the interim, allergy shots should be considered for patients with asthma who fit the criteria specified above if their allergic history and skin test results correlate, and if there is a reasonable chance of success with shots for the specific allergen in question.

Allergy shots are most effective for the seasonal pollens and dust. Although shots are not a cure, they can help to reduce your symptoms and your need for medication. There is no objective measure of the success of allergy shots except a comparison of your past and present allergic histories. Success with allergy shots for hay fever caused by the seasonal pollens is as high as 85 percent; the rate of success with dust is somewhat less, approximately 70 percent, undoubtedly reflecting the fact that dust is made up of so many different components. The success rate for the molds is more variable.

The Allergy Shot Program. Once the decision has been made to begin a program of allergy shots, a serum is prepared containing purified, sterile extracts of the allergens that correspond to your allergic history and skin test results. The serum does not contain any medication. The serum is then diluted three to four times to create bottles of varying strengths, so as to gradually adjust your body to receiving the allergens.

Allergy shots are given initially at weekly or biweekly intervals, starting with the weakest serum and proceeding to the strongest serum. The shots are given on a year-round basis. The dose is gradually increased each week, providing that there are no adverse reactions. Once the build-up process has been completed (which usually takes from several months to one year), the highest dose (called the maintenance dose) is given initially once a week, then every other week, and eventually every four weeks. Improvement in allergy symptoms is usually noted between the first and second years by patients who have reached the higher doses. If allergy shots have proved to be of benefit during the first two years, the shots are typically continued for a three to five-year period.

Risks of Allergy Shots. The most common reaction to an allergy shot is swelling along with redness and itchiness at the site of the injection. This type of reaction usually goes away on its own although, on occasion, the use of ice and an antihistamine may be necessary to reduce the swelling. However, swelling at the shot site is an important observation and should be reported to your allergist. The swelling may suggest that the dose of the allergy shot needs to be reduced with the next shot. If the swelling is larger than a quarter, the dosage of the next injection must be reduced, as this may be a clue that a more serious reaction could occur if the dose is increased.

The most serious reaction from an allergy shot is called anaphylaxis. If this reaction were to occur, it would typically begin within twenty minutes after the allergy shot. Since severe anaphylactic reactions can be life threatening, all allergy shots should be given in the presence of a physician experienced in treating anaphylaxis, and you should remain in the doctor's office for a full fifteen to twenty minutes after each injection. Indications that you may be having a more serious reaction include an increase in your allergy symptoms (such as itchy eyes, nasal stuffiness, and sneezing), difficulty breathing (due to increased asthma symptoms), difficulty swallowing, or the sensation of passing out. Redness of the face and itchiness of the skin often accompany these symptoms. The pulse rate increases and the blood pressure can drop. An injection of Adrenalin and antihistamines (such as Benadryl) are usually given to counter these reactions. This is often sufficient but more intensive medication may be necessary.

Fortunately, the chances of an anaphylactic reaction are small. However, if you experience any of the above symptoms after getting an allergy shot, you should report this to your doctor at once. Never leave your doctor's office if you do not feel just right. Also, be sure to report all symptoms that you experienced after your last allergy shot to the doctor or nurse before the next one is given.

Newer Allergy Shot Programs (Not Yet Approved) Offer Less Risk of Reactions and Faster Relief. As mentioned above, allergens currently used for immunotherapy carry the risk of causing allergic reactions when administered in high dose. In order to reduce the risk of reaction, the shot program starts at low doses with close observation for signs indicating a greater chance of reaction (such as swelling at the shot site). Newer developments have altered the allergen that is injected so that it carries a reduced chance of causing reactions and therefore can be administered in higher doses more rapidly. There is the hope that with these new allergens, called polymerized allergens, the benefits noted after years of allergy shots possibly can be achieved, with reduced risk of reaction, after a dozen or so shots. Preliminary studies of these newer shots are promising for grasses and ragweed. As yet, polymerized allergens have not yet been approved by the Food and Drug Administration.

Should Allergy Shots Be Part of an Asthma Treatment Plan? If allergy is clearly one of the factors that precipitates your asthma symptoms (as confirmed by positive allergy skin tests), allergy shots should be considered if they are recommended by your allergist, especially if you fit the description of candidacy for allergy shots presented earlier. If successful, the results from allergy shots can be truly remarkable, as many patients are free of symptoms during pollen seasons once the higher doses of the shots have been reached. Most patients are pleased if they notice that they have less symptoms and are able to reduce their need for medication. This is a realistic goal of an allergy shot program. As medications simply hide your allergy symptoms, the potential of reducing or possibly eliminating your symptoms with allergy shots should not be overlooked. For best results, you should consult a doctor who has been trained in the field of allergy, preferably an allergist certified by the American Academy of Allergy and Clinical Immunology. See also Appendix B (page 345).

QUESTIONS

1. Should I continue to take my allergy medications even though I have started getting allergy shots?
Yes. As it takes from several months to one year to pro-

gress to high dose allergy shots, allergy medications are often needed even though a program of allergy shots has been started. Remember that allergy shots do not contain medication. Rather, allergy serum contains small doses of the allergens that correspond to your allergy history and skin testing. The eventual goal with allergy shots is to reduce your need for medications and to reduce your symptoms. However, this does take time, with a noticeable response usually seen between the first and second year of allergy shots.

2. I know people who have been getting allergy shots for years and years. Is that the usual case?

No. An allergy shot program usually is for a three- to five-year period, depending on your response to the shots. If you have had good results with the shots, and if you have been comfortable during your symptomatic time period for two years, the shots may be discontinued. Most patients will be able to stop the shots without a worsening of symptoms. However, some patients will require a "refresher" program of shots after several years. In addition, there are some patients who do not respond to the allergy shots even in proper dosages.

3. Are there any long-term risks associated with allergy shots?

To date, there do not appear to be any significant long-term risks with allergy shots for most individuals. There does not appear to be any increased risk of cancer (a question asked by many patients). Clearly, the greatest risk associated with allergy shots is that of anaphylaxis—an immediate, severe, potentially life-threatening reaction following an allergy shot. Fortunately, this is a rare occurrence and can usually be managed with Adrenalin in the doctor's office.

4. I have asthma that flares during the ragweed season. I have trouble tolerating the asthma medications my doctor has prescribed for me. Even though I don't have hay fever, could allergy shots help?

Yes, if your allergy skin testing matches your allergic history. However, allergy shots must be taken on a year-round basis even though you have symptoms only during the ragweed season. Therefore, it would be a good idea to discuss with your doctor whether there are any medications that can be tried in place of the medications you are now using. The rate of success with ragweed allergy shots is quite good. Many allergists find that allergy shots in high dose are as effective in helping to control asthma symptoms as in controlling hay fever symptoms. However, definitive studies necessary to substantiate this observation are just now getting under way.

5. If my asthma is well managed with medications alone, why should I bother with allergy shots?

This may be a personal decision but it should be made with complete understanding of the potential benefit of allergy shots. Medications used in asthma management simply help to control asthma symptoms—unfortunately, the available medications do not offer a cure. If your asthma history points to an allergic explanation for your asthma flares, allergy shots should be considered, as they offer the possibility of reducing and perhaps eliminating the need for asthma medication and reducing your asthma symptoms. Allergy shots are not appropriate for all asthma patients, but when appropriate, they can bring about noteworthy improvement.

6. After every allergy shot I get a lump the size of a golf ball. It goes away by the next day. Should I mention this to my doctor?

Absolutely. It is important that you relay to your doctor all information concerning swelling at the shot site, so that appropriate dosing alterations can be made. Local swelling that increases in size with each stronger allergy shot indicates that you may be at risk for a more serious reaction. So be sure to tell your doctor so that you can continue to receive your allergy shots safely.

7. I am allergic to cats. Every time I am around a cat, I start to wheeze. Should I take allergy shots for cats?

As cats can be avoided, this is always the preferable first step approach. If your cat has access to your bedroom, preventing this is often sufficient. If you cannot avoid being exposed to cats, allergy shots can be considered, although somewhat reluctantly, since there is a greater risk of large local and systemic reactions with shots for cat allergy. New allergens for cat desensitization are being developed that may offer greater success with less reactivity.

8. I prefer to have my sister, who is a registered nurse, give me my allergy shots at home as opposed to getting them at the allergist's office. Is there any reason why this is not acceptable?

Allergy shots are best given in the presence of a physician who is able to manage anaphylaxis should it occur, especially since there may be a need for medications in addition to Adrenalin. Although severe reactions are rare, every allergy shot must still be taken seriously. Allergy shots in high dosages should always be given with a doctor present.

SUMMARY: ALLERGY IMMUNOTHERAPY (SHOTS)

1. Allergy shots are small doses of the allergen(s) to which you are sensitive. Allergy shots do not contain medications.

2. Allergy shots reduce your sensitivity over time to the injected allergen. Improvement is usually noted between the first and second year of treatment. The allergy shot program usually is for a three- to five-year period.

3. Allergy shots are not right for every asthma patient—as a first step, your allergic history and skin test results must support each other. Accurate assessment of the role of allergy in your asthma is essential.

4. Allergy shots are most effective for the seasonal pollens and dust. Shots for allergy to molds are less consistently successful. Since there is an increased risk of adverse reactions with allergy shots using animal dander, avoidance of animals is preferable to allergy shots for this type of allergy.

5. The risks associated with allergy shots range from swelling at the shot site to more generalized reactions such as anaphylaxis, which is potentially life threatening. Fortunately, the risk of anaphylaxis is small, but it emphasizes the importance of receiving your allergy injections in the presence of a doctor and waiting a full fifteen to twenty minutes after each injection for observation. Notify your doctor of any adverse reactions following an allergy shot, including swelling at the shot site of greater than a quarter in size, as a reduction in the dosage of the injection may be necessary.

6. Newer allergy shots, using allergens that have been altered (polymerized) to reduce the risk of adverse reactions so that a more rapid dosage build-up can be accomplished, are not yet available but offer a promising outlook.

7. The goal with allergy shots is to reduce your need for medications and to reduce your symptoms. It is unwise to think of allergy shots as a total cure for your allergies, although this does happen for some people. Medications simply hide your allergy symptoms, but allergy shots offer the potential of more permanent relief if the allergic contribution to your asthma is clear-cut.

PART THREE

◇◇◇◇◇

Asthma in Special Circumstances

◇ **8** ◇

Asthma in Children

Asthma is a leading cause of illness in children, accounting for over 20 percent of missed school days in this country. Asthma touches many aspects of the child's and the family's life. Asthma can limit the child's time to exercise and to be with friends; it can necessitate daily medications, as well as emergency visits to the doctor or the hospital. Clearly, asthma can have impact on the psychological well-being of both the child and the family.

In view of these possibilities, it is especially important that childhood asthma be well managed. You should be fully informed about your child's asthma, and make certain that you understand the reasoning behind your child's asthma management program. When problems arise, you should keep in close contact with your child's asthma doctor. Many of the points previously discussed with regard to ideal asthma management hold true during childhood. Those points that distinguish asthma in children from asthma in adults will be discussed in this chapter.

Statistics Concerning the Frequency and Typical Course of Asthma During Childhood. It is estimated that somewhere between 5 and 10 percent of children in the United States have asthma symptoms at some point while growing up. The actual percentage may be even higher since asthma symptoms can take many forms, such as a subtle cough, that may never be diagnosed as asthma.

But a few things can be said with certainty: (a) Asthma and allergies are the most common chronic problem in children under age seventeen. (b) Asthma is the most common cause of school absenteeism of the chronic illnesses affecting children in the United States.(c) Asthma is one of the most frequent, if not the most frequent, reason for children to be admitted to a hospital. (d) Asthma is more common in children than in adults, although asthma can occur at any age.

Boys Are More Likely Than Girls to Have Asthma During Childhood. Statistics show that in children under ten years of age, asthma is twice as likely to occur in boys as in girls. The reason for this difference is not yet understood. As children approach adolescence, the ratio of boys to girls with asthma is about the same.

Age at Which Asthma Begins. Asthma can occur at any age but is more likely to occur within the first five years of life. When asthma develops during childhood, allergies are usually a contributing factor. However, as with all age groups, it is possible for children to have asthma and not be allergic.

Many Children "Outgrow" Asthma. As a child gets older and the size of the airways increases, asthma symptoms are likely to improve or disappear. Approximately 50 percent of all children with asthma are free of symptoms by the age of fifteen. However, there are no fixed rules, and asthma remissions and flares can occur at any time during childhood or adulthood. Although children who have persistent daily symptoms are more likely to continue to have asthma symptoms beyond childhood, there is no way of predicting which children will continue to have asthma symptoms into adulthood.

Factors that seem to favor persistence of asthma beyond childhood include: (a) asthma that begins at less than two years of age; (b) allergy as a contributing factor; (c) presence of nasal polyps (see page 299); (d) gender, with boys being at a greater risk; and (e) frequent asthma attacks or routine wheezing that is difficult to manage. Children who wheeze only when they have upper respiratory infections are thought to be more likely to "outgrow" asthma symptoms.

As previously mentioned, asthma has no permanent damaging effect on the lungs or airways. Asthma does not lead to emphysema.

Risk Factors for Developing Asthma. Clearly, heredity plays a major role in the tendency to develop asthma. The genetic mode of transmission probably involves many factors. The tendency to develop asthma is not as simple as, for example, the tendency to have brown or blue eyes. Although the chances of developing asthma can be influenced by various factors (such as allergies, infections, irritants, and environment), the genetic tendency for asthma in all probability must first be present. Infections such as croup and bronchiolitis (page 209) seem to increase the tendency toward asthma. In addition, cigarette smoking by parents has been implicated as a potential factor for increasing the risk that children with the tendency to develop asthma will suffer asthma symptoms, as lower breathing test results have been observed in children whose parents are smokers.

Factors That Cause Asthma Symptoms. The initial section of this book provides a comprehensive review of the factors that can trigger asthma symptoms. These same factors can contribute to asthma in children. You must determine which of the factors seems to affect your child's asthma, so that you can be prepared for situations when asthma symptoms are likely to flare. A clear understanding of exercise-induced asthma is important as it is common during childhood. A comprehensive approach to the problem of exercise-induced asthma is worthwhile in view of the importance of exercise for children.

Asthma Symptoms Can Vary. Asthma symptoms are not limited to wheezing, and can be as commonplace as a hacky, persistent cough. Since some children are able to tolerate asthma symptoms and continue to play as if there were no problem, parents should learn to recognize when subtle asthma symptoms might possibly be occurring. It is also important to know that wheezing may *not* be heard when asthma is severe, as there may not be enough air movement through the airways to produce a wheezing sound. You should not allow your child's asthma symptoms to progress to that point.

Problems During Childhood That Can Mimic Asthma. Every child with asthma should be under the ongoing care of a doctor who routinely takes care of asthma patients. The doctor should see your child several times when he or she is having asthma symptoms in order to evaluate the frequency, severity, and possible precipitants of the symptoms, and determine appropriate therapy. During these visits with the doctor, you should become familiar with the medications recommended for your child and be certain that your questions are answered. This time period also gives the doctor the opportunity to confirm his initial diagnosis. Although the diagnosis of asthma is usually quite straightforward, several medical problems can at times masquerade as asthma, making the correct diagnosis more complicated.

The list of problems that can mimic asthma symptoms is extensive. Some of them include croup, bronchitis, bronchiolitis, congenital abnormalities of the upper airway (throat), gastroesophageal reflux (see page 282), foreign bodies, and cystic fibrosis. Needless to say, you are counting on your doctor for the correct diagnosis. If you feel uncomfortable about the diagnosis, discuss this with your doctor, as a second opinion can be reassuring.

Croup. Croup is a viral illness which usually occurs after the child has had an upper respiratory infection. In children under the age of five, croup often begins with nighttime hoarseness and a barking cough that comes from the throat. Another symptom of croup is difficulty inhaling (as opposed to difficulty exhaling typically seen with asthma). Any symptoms that mimic croup, cause difficulty breathing, or differ from your child's ordinary asthma symptoms should be reported to your child's doctor immediately.

Bronchitis. Bronchitis means inflammation of the air tubes (the bronchi). Generally this occurs as a result of an infection, typically a viral infection. Often it is difficult to distinguish bronchitis from asthma. The term "asthmatic bronchitis" is used when an infection triggers asthma symptoms. With bronchitis, usually the child first has nasal congestion and a runny nose, then a slight fever and a cough along with asthmalike symptoms. Often by treating asthma symptoms as well as the bronchitis, there is marked improvement.

Bronchiolitis. Bronchiolitis, which occurs in infants and very young children, is a viral respiratory infection. It causes a runny nose, coughing, and wheezing. The difficulty in breathing may be severe and the baby usually looks quite ill. These symptoms are often difficult to distinguish from asthma. As high as 50 percent of children who have had bronchiolitis go on to have asthma symptoms in later childhood.

Obstruction of the Upper Airway. Partial blockage of the upper airway can give rise to asthmalike symptoms. For example, heavy secretions in the upper airway can cause the infant's breathing to mimic the wheezing sounds of asthma. Another condition in infants that can cause asthmalike symptoms is called stridor. In this case, the soft cartilage in the infant's throat causes a harsh noise to emanate from the throat and sometimes from the chest. A thorough evaluation by a doctor familiar with asthma or by an ear, nose, and throat doctor (otolaryngologist) should reveal any upper airway abnormalities.

Acute Epiglottitis. By far the most serious of problems of the upper airway is acute epiglottitis. This illness is usually caused by a bacterial infection from the organism Haemophilus influenzae. Acute epiglottitis usually begins rapidly, with high fever, sore throat, and difficulty in breathing and swallowing. If the swallowing is quite difficult, the child drools. Acute epiglottitis is a serious, potentially life-threatening condition which requires immediate medical attention in order to ensure that the airway is kept open. If your child has any of these signs, you should immediately contact your pediatrician or proceed to the emergency room.

Foreign Bodies. Foreign bodies such as peas, peanuts, or small objects can become lodged in a child's airways or lungs and cause coughing and wheezing, which at times can be mistaken for asthma symptoms. An X-ray examination of the chest may not detect the presence of foreign bodies such as these. It is possible for the foreign material to remain in the lung and trigger intermittent chest symptoms. Foreign bodies must be removed by passing a tube into the lung to prevent damage to the lung.

Cystic Fibrosis. Cystic fibrosis is a genetically transmitted disease primarily affecting Caucasians. The incidence of cystic fibrosis is approximately one in every two thousand live births. This disease involves the pancreas as well as the lungs. Deficiencies in the pancreas caused by cystic fibrosis result in diarrhea and a failure to thrive during infancy despite a good appetite. Bulky, foul-smelling stools are frequent. Chest symptoms occur as a result of blockage of the airways caused by thick mucus secretions, and are further complicated by infections. Patients with cystic fibrosis experience wheezing that can mimic the wheezing of asthma. They can also have typical allergy symptoms and positive allergy skin tests. Nasal polyps are often present as well (see page 299). Some patients with cystic fibrosis have lung problems but exhibit no other symptoms for some time, making the diagnosis more deceptive. In order to determine if someone has cystic fibrosis, an analysis is often made of the amount of chloride in the person's sweat. The chloride level is elevated in the perspiration of a person with cystic fibrosis. This test is often performed on children who have chronic lung problems to determine whether cystic fibrosis is present.

Treatment of Asthma in Children. Although asthma cannot be cured, it can be well managed. The goal of asthma management is to allow your child to live as normally as children who do not have asthma, with a medication program that is as easy to use and as free of side effects as possible.

As discussed in Chapter 3, the three approaches to treating asthma are the avoidance of known allergens and irritants, the use of medications, and a program of allergy immunotherapy (shots). Each of these areas will be addressed to highlight the points that distinguish management of childhood asthma from adult asthma management.

Avoidance Techniques. You should first be certain that you are familiar with the factors that precipitate asthma symptoms in your child (see Chapter 2). If allergy is one of the factors, changes in your child's environmental exposures can be truly worthwhile. You should strive in particular to make your child's bedroom a haven from allergic exposure. This can greatly reduce asthma symptoms in some children, since your child probably spends at least eight to ten hours in the bedroom each night. Avoidance of pets (especially when they sleep in the child's bed), stuffed animals, and feather pillows can greatly improve asthma symptoms. Although the steps for reducing dust and mold exposure may be somewhat inconvenient, these suggestions should be given serious attention if your child is allergic to dust and mold (see page 189).

It is also important to review any irritants that in the past have triggered asthma symptoms. For example, if smoke, perfumes, and newsprint cause your child's asthma to flare, exposure to these irritants should be avoided whenever possible. In addition, you should know in advance the steps to take if your child does become exposed to an irritant and begins to have asthma symptoms. In such a situation, your child should leave the area, use the medication prescribed for sudden asthma symptoms (such as an inhaled or oral Adrenalin-like bronchodilator), and stay calm and await any improvement in symptoms. If symptoms do not improve, use a back-up medication and notify your child's asthma doctor.

Medications Used in Asthma Management for Children. Chapter 3 discusses each of the medications currently used in asthma management. This section highlights points that pertain to children.

Adrenalin and Adrenalin-like Medications. Adrenalin (epinephrine) given by injection is by far the most commonly used medication for treating asthma flares in children. It is often used in the doctor's office or in the emergency room to bring an asthma attack under control. For children who are already taking asthma medications, Adrenalin is used if the prescribed back-up medications have not brought relief. Adrenalin is administered by injection just under the skin (subcutaneously). It is preferable to have a doctor present when Adrenalin is given, since Adrenalin will increase your child's heart rate and may cause shakiness, nausea, and vomiting. You should also be aware that your child will probably look quite pale after receiving an Adrenalin injection. Once the Adrenalin brings asthma symptoms under control, many doctors will inject a long-acting Adrenalin-like preparation called Sus-Phrine to keep asthma symptoms under control until oral medications such as theophylline have time to work.

If prescribed by your doctor, Adrenalin can be administered at home for attacks that are frequent and severe. However, with the availability of nebulizers for home use, it is now rarely necessary to give an Adrenalin shot at home. A nebulizer can be most helpful in bringing a severe asthma episode under control, since it provides an easy method for a child to use a quick-acting bronchodilating medication such as metaproterenol (Metaprel or Alupent) or isoetharine (Bronkosol). Many of the companies that sell nebulizers employ trained respiratory technicians who will bring the nebulizer to your home and teach you how to use it in accordance with the doctor's instructions. If this service is not available, ask your child's doctor to show you how to administer properly a breathing treatment with a nebulizer.

If Adrenalin is frequently needed to control asthma symptoms, this indicates that your child's medication program is insufficient or that the attacks are quite severe. Be prepared for subsequent attacks so that hopefully you will not have to rush to the doctor's office or the emergency room for Adrenalin. The simplest approach is to use a bronchodilating inhaler, which can offer relief within minutes when used properly (see page 68).

For children under the age of six, who often are unable to

master proper inhaler technique, there are two alternatives:
(1) use of an inhalation chamber, whereby the medication
from the bronchodilating inhaler is sprayed into the chamber
and the child simply takes a big breath from the mouthpiece
of the chamber, with no need to activate the inhaler properly;
and (2) use of an oral Adrenalin-like bronchodilator such as
metaproterenol (Metaprel or Alupent) or albuterol (Proventil
or Ventolin) which is taken in pill or liquid form and works
within fifteen to thirty minutes.

As a back-up to these Adrenalin-like medications, a short-
acting product that contains theophylline should also be available. If the back-up medication proves unrewarding in halting
asthma symptoms, promptly notify your child's asthma doctor. At that point it may well be necessary for your child to
be treated at the doctor's office or in the emergency room.

Theophylline Products. Theophylline is frequently used
in managing asthma in children who have symptoms on a
daily basis. Because it is an oral medication, available as a
liquid as well as in the form of pills and capsules, it is acceptable for use in all age groups when taken in the proper
dose. One method of administering theophylline is in a
"sprinkle" form, whereby capsules containing theophylline
are designed to be opened and the contents mixed into food
such as apple sauce.

Interestingly, children from ages one to twelve have the
tendency to break down theophylline rapidly within their bodies. Thus, children in this age group tend to need higher
dosages of theophylline per kilogram of body weight than
adults. Infants need lower doses than children over one year
of age. Children over the age of twelve often need less theophylline than they needed at a younger age. Theophylline
dosages should therefore be reassessed intermittently
throughout childhood by use of a theophylline blood test to
ensure that the dose is within a safe range.

When a child's asthma cannot be controlled using the standard recommended theophylline dose, it is then necessary to
determine the exact dosage of theophylline present in the
child's blood. A blood test called a theophylline level is performed to determine the exact amount of theophylline in your

child's bloodstream at the time the test is given. This test allows the doctor to determine whether the child's dose of theophylline can be elevated without increasing the risk of theophylline side effects. When the blood theophylline level is maintained within the range of 10 to 20 micrograms of theophylline per milliliter of blood serum, most patients will achieve the greatest benefit from theophylline with the least risk of side effects. This is called the therapeutic range. As the level begins to approach 15 to 20, patients sometimes notice headache, nausea, vomiting, or diarrhea. The most severe side effect of theophylline is seizure; fortunately this is quite rare when the dose of theophylline is kept within the standard therapeutic range.

Some children will experience theophylline side effects such as nausea or headache even when the dose of theophylline is within the standard therapeutic range. In addition, some children develop behavioral problems at school and at home due to the restlessness triggered by this medication. Children taking theophylline sometimes have trouble falling asleep and, as a result, are often sleepy at school. If you notice or suspect any of these problems, you should mention this to your doctor. The theophylline dose can then be reduced, or the timing of the doses changed so that the theophylline does not reach its peak when the child is trying to fall asleep. With these adjustments in your child's use of theophylline, additional asthma medications may be necessary to assist in controlling asthma symptoms.

Review of the section on theophylline, beginning on page 78, is important. You should be familiar with those medications that can cause the level of the theophylline in your child's blood to rise or fall (see page 90). For example, the antibiotic erythromycin can cause the theophylline level to increase. Therefore, your child's dosage of theophylline needs to be reduced when your child is taking this antibiotic. With this background, you will understand why it may sometimes be necessary for your child's doctor to make temporary adjustments in your child's theophylline dose.

Cromolyn Sodium. Cromolyn sodium (Intal) is one of the most frequently overlooked asthma medications. Yet it can be a truly beneficial medication for children who have routine asthma symptoms. Cromolyn is a preventative medication and not a bronchodilator. It is used to prevent asthma symptoms rather than to treat asthma symptoms once they occur. With this in mind and with an appropriate treatment program to turn to if asthma flares, cromolyn is worthy of consideration, as it can often provide excellent results.

Cromolyn must be inhaled, as it is not well absorbed into the body from the gastrointestinal tract when it is swallowed. Cromolyn is available in powder form for use with a spinhaler, in liquid form for use in a nebulizer, and just recently in inhaler form. The nebulizer is ideal for use by children under the age of six for whom it might be difficult to use a spinhaler. It is often helpful to use a bronchodilating inhaler such as albuterol (Proventil or Ventolin) before using cromolyn, to open the airways and allow the cromolyn better access to the airways. For children unable to use an inhaler, a bronchodilating solution such as metaproterenol can be used prior to or along with cromolyn in a nebulizer.

Cromolyn is usually taken three to four times a day. As cromolyn can prevent asthma triggered by exercise, the daytime doses of cromolyn are often scheduled twenty minutes before exercise.

Cromolyn is essentially free of side effects, and does not usually cause personality change or restlessness. It is a good choice for children who have frequent asthma symptoms and are intolerant of the side effects of theophylline. The most common side effect of cromolyn is minor irritation of the throat due to the lactose base of the medication. Severe reactions to cromolyn are rare but have been reported in isolated cases (see Chapter 3). To date, it appears that cromolyn can be used quite safely by most children, with little concern for side effects.

Steroids. All of the principles discussed in Chapter 3 are pertinent to the use of steroids by children. When asthma symptoms are out of control and fail to respond to the backup measures outlined in your management plan, your doctor should be notified promptly. *IT WOULD BE A MISTAKE TO*

WITHHOLD STEROIDS DURING AN ACUTE, DIFFICULT-TO-MANAGE ASTHMA FLARE OUT OF CONCERN FOR STEROID SIDE EFFECTS, especially since serious side effects are usually not associated with short-term use. In addition, it is faulty reasoning to think that using steroids for a few days will make your child forever dependent on steroids. Needless to say, it is preferable if children as well as adults can avoid using steroids. However, when asthma is out of control, the benefits of using steroids far outweigh the risks.

Steroids are the last medication that should be added to a routine asthma medication program. The possibility of reducing the steroid dose by using alternative medications should be considered at all times when a child is taking steroids. If there is no alternative to steroids and they are required on a routine basis, they should be taken in as ideal a manner as possible (see page 110).

Steroids that are inhaled are less likely to cause steroid side effects than steroids taken daily by mouth. For children over the age of five who routinely require oral steroids, it is often possible to replace or reduce the dose by using an inhaled steroid such as beclomethasone (Vanceril or Beclovent). For children under five years of age who routinely need steroids, a liquid form of steroid that could be inhaled via a nebulizer would be ideal; unfortunately, this is not yet available. As an alternative to steroids taken orally for the child in this age group, steroids that can be inhaled through the use of an inhalation chamber can be tried (see page 70).

For children who are unable to swallow pills, the steroid prednisone is available in liquid form (Liquid Pred Syrup). Each teaspoon contains 5 milligrams of prednisone. If you do not have the liquid prednisone preparation but do have prednisone in pill form, the pills can be crushed and given to the child in food such as apple sauce or chocolate syrup. Your child's doctor will advise you of the proper dosage of steroid and the appropriate timing of the dose. All instructions for the use of steroids must be carefully followed.

You should be aware of the potential side effects associated with long-term steroid use. These are reviewed in detail in Chapter 19. One steroid side effect that is of great concern in children is growth retardation, as it may not be reversible.

Routine follow-up care by your child's doctor, with emphasis on the proper use of the prescribed medications, should allow the steroid dose to be the least amount necessary to control asthma symptoms.

Allergy Immunotherapy (Shots). Allergy shots can be quite helpful in managing asthma during childhood if your child's allergy history is supported by his skin test results. Namely, if your child has a history of asthma flares in the spring or fall, and his allergy tests are clearly positive to allergens that are present in the environment during that time period, allergy shots should be considered. When allergy shots are given for nasal problems, they have been shown to reduce the need for medication and reduce the frequency of asthma symptoms. Allergy shots tend to work especially well for the seasonal pollens when given properly at high doses. Patients who are sensitive to ragweed achieve especially good results from allergy shots, with a success rate as high as 85 percent. Although to date there have been few clear-cut scientific studies concerning allergy shots for asthma because of the difficulty in designing such studies, allergists have for years noted improvements when shots are administered to properly selected patients. A full discussion of allergy shots is presented on page 194.

Complications of Childhood Asthma. By far the most common complication of childhood asthma is infection. Viral (as opposed to bacterial) are the most common types of infection to trigger a worsening of asthma symptoms. Often additional asthma medications are needed during the first few days of a viral infection. Antibiotics will not help fight off viral infections. However, during a prolonged asthma flare, an antibiotic is often given to be sure that the mucus trapped in the airways has not become infected by bacteria (which is responsive to an antibiotic). Although viral infections are more common precipitants of asthma flares, the possibility of bacterial infections (including strep throat) should not be overlooked. If mucus from the child's nose or chest is green or yellow in color (rather than clear), consideration can be given to the use of an antibiotic. If the antibiotic erythromycin is prescribed, the child's theophylline dosage must be reduced.

Other complications of childhood asthma can include: (a) atelectasis, collapse of a portion of the lung as a result of extensive mucus plugging the airway; (b) pneumothorax, the presence of free air within the chest that has escaped from the airways; and (c) cough syncope, extensive coughing resulting in fainting, with recovery within minutes. If there is any change in your child's asthma symptoms, especially increased shortness of breath in association with chest or neck pain, your child's asthma doctor should be notified.

Growth retardation can occur with difficult-to-manage asthma. In rare cases this has been reported even in children who have not taken steroids. Your child's doctor needs to follow closely the child's height on a growth chart, so that any drop-off from the normal growth pattern can be recognized. In addition, severe childhood asthma can result in a deformity of the chest wall called pseudorachitic deformity. Fortunately, both of these complications are quite rare, but they emphasize the importance of early asthma management.

Patient Education Is Essential. The goal of asthma therapy is to allow your child to live as normally as possible. To achieve this goal, you cannot be a passive bystander. It is essential that both you and your child understand asthma and the medications that have been recommended to manage the problem. Of late there has been great emphasis placed by the medical community on the importance of patient education, and this is rightfully so. One example is the Asthma Care Training (ACT) program developed through the Asthma and Allergy Foundation of America, which teaches children how to recognize their asthma symptoms and to take the lead in following their doctors' instructions. Other sources of information about patient education are presented in Appendix B. Under the direction of your physician, a program that allows your child to take part in his asthma management will give both you and your child the confidence that the problem is under control, and that his asthma makes him no different from other children.

SUMMARY: ASTHMA IN CHILDREN

1. Of the chronic childhood illnesses, asthma accounts for
    the greatest number of missed school days in the United
    States. When asthma symptoms are frequent and give
    rise to emergency visits to the doctor or hospital, the
    impact on the child and family can be significant. Asthma
    care should not be limited to the administration of med-
    ications, but should also strive to secure the emotional
    well-being of the child and family.

2. The estimate of the number of children in the United
    States affected by asthma is between 5 and 10 percent.
    Asthma is the most common chronic (long-term) medical
    problem affecting children under the age of seventeen.

3. Asthma can occur at any age but is more common in
    children than in adults. In children under the age of ten,
    boys are more likely to have asthma than girls.

4. Approximately 50 percent of all children with asthma do
    "outgrow" it by age fifteen. A contributing factor is the
    increase in the size of the airways as the child matures.
    Since the tendency toward asthma usually still exists,
    asthma symptoms can recur at any time throughout life.
    If asthma symptoms have occurred on a daily basis dur-
    ing childhood, they are more likely to persist beyond the
    teenage years.

5. Heredity determines whether a person has the potential
    for developing asthma. Factors such as the environment,
    infections, and allergies undoubtedly play a role in
    whether asthma in fact develops.

6. Asthma symptoms can vary and are not limited to
    wheezing. A persistent cough may well be a sign of sub-
    tle asthma symptoms.

7. Croup, bronchitis, congenital abnormalities of the upper
    airway, and other problems can mimic asthma symp-

toms. Several follow-up visits with your doctor may be necessary in order to clarify the diagnosis. The most serious of these problems is cystic fibrosis, which can be diagnosed with a test measuring sweat chlorides.

8. Treatment of asthma in children is similar to treatment of adults with asthma, and includes avoidance of offending allergens and irritants, judicious use of medication and, when appropriate, a program of allergy shots.

9. An asthma management plan for children should consider: (a) proper adjustment of the theophylline dose—because children from ages one to twelve have the tendency to break down theophylline rapidly, they usually require relatively more theophylline than adults, and their blood theophylline level should be checked intermittently during childhood to be sure that the dose is correct; (b) a plan for managing sudden asthma flares—this will often include an oral, rapidly acting Adrenalin-like bronchodilator in liquid form, such as metaproterenol (Alupent or Metaprel), and/or the use of a home nebulizer to administer a bronchodilating solution, especially for children under the age of six, who usually have difficulty mastering inhaler technique; (c) the use of an inhalation chamber by children who are unable to use an inhaler properly, in order to take advantage of the rapidly acting bronchodilating inhalers; (d) the use of preventative medications such as cromolyn sodium (Intal), which is essentially free of side effects and is available in liquid form for use with a nebulizer (ideal for small children), in powder form for use in a spinhaler, and just recently in inhaler form.

10. Steroids are the last medication choice for routine use. Steroids should never be withheld during an acute, difficult-to-manage asthma flare out of concern for steroid side effects or future dependency on steroids. The potential for steroid side effects is associated with their long-term, not their short-term, use.

11. Allergy shots can be helpful in managing asthma when a child's allergy skin test results are supported by his or her medical history. Improvement in asthma symptoms from allergy shots has been observed by doctors for years, but has not been confirmed by a clear-cut scientific study because of the difficulty in designing such a study.

12. Severe childhood asthma can in rare cases lead to growth retardation, even in children who have not used steroids. Since the use of steroids can increase the likelihood of growth retardation, the necessity for steroids and the steroid dose should be reassessed on a frequent basis.

13. Both the child and the parents must be well informed in order for asthma care to be successful.

◇ 9 ◇

Asthma and Pregnancy

The overall incidence of asthma during pregnancy is somewhere between 0.4 and 1.3 percent. Naturally, the risk of
asthma during pregnancy is greater for women who had
asthma before becoming pregnant. Therefore, it is important
to understand the effect of pregnancy on asthma, the effect
of asthma on pregnancy, and the currently accepted approach
for the use of necessary asthma medications during pregnancy.

Effects of Pregnancy on Asthma. As a rule of thumb,
one third of all pregnant asthma patients have asthma symptoms that improve during pregnancy, one third have symptoms that remain the same, and one third have symptoms that
become worse. More than half of those women whose asthma
symptoms were worse during their first pregnancy will probably have similar symptoms with subsequent pregnancies.
Typically, the women who have worse symptoms during pregnancy are those women who have more difficult asthma;
namely, those women who require steroids and who have frequent asthma flares tend to be worse during pregnancy. Needless to say, there are exceptions to these observations.
Therefore, every asthma patient who becomes pregnant

should be carefully followed by the doctor who manages her asthma, as well as her obstetrician.

Effects of Asthma on Pregnancy. The older medical literature is somewhat unclear as to the effect of asthma on the mother and fetus. However, recent studies suggest that, in general, asthma in a mother whose asthma is well managed and is free of complications imposes no increased risk for either the mother or the fetus. However, some questions still remain unanswered, such as: (a) whether the incidence of premature births is slightly higher for women with asthma than for the general population; (b) which, if any, of the potential asthma complications may have impact on the well-being of the fetus; and (c) whether there is any prenatal test that can indicate the chance of the fetus developing asthma.

Asthma Medications During Pregnancy. Asthma management during pregnancy differs little from routine asthma management. Of course, it would be best if your asthma could be managed during pregnancy without the need for medications. Since this is often not the case, you should review your medication program with your doctor to be certain that your usual medications are acceptable.

It is important to be aware that the benefit of asthma medications in keeping your asthma under control needs to be weighted against the potential risk of side effects to your baby. The *Physicians' Desk Reference (PDR)*, which most physicians rely upon for information concerning the acceptability of various medications during pregnancy, is often of little help in this regard. For many asthma medications the *PDR* simply indicates that safety in pregnancy has not been established. In many cases this caution does not imply that the medication has been found to be unsafe during pregnancy. Rather, this often indicates that an acceptable medical study has not been performed, due to the difficulty of designing such a study with pregnant asthma patients.

Fortunately, experience has shown that, to date, theophylline and several of the inhaled and oral Adrenalin-like bronchodilators can be used during pregnancy with little risk to the fetus. Steroids are also acceptable during pregnancy when there is no alternative; recent studies have shown that there is no increased risk of congenital abnormalities in the fetus, negating the major concern in the past for an increased risk of cleft palate.

Appropriately selected medications should be used to control asthma during pregnancy when necessary, as inadequately controlled asthma can be dangerous for both the mother and the fetus.

Theophylline. Complications associated with theophylline taken in proper dosage during pregnancy are infrequent. When oral medications are necessary to control asthma during pregnancy, theophylline should be the mainstay in most cases. Before adding another medication, the level of theophylline in the blood should be checked to be certain that the theophylline dose is optimal. During pregnancy it is especially important that the theophylline dose is not too high, as this could increase the risk of side effects such as nausea, diarrhea, and headache. As discussed earlier, there is no standard dose of theophylline that is correct for everyone. The dose of theophylline must be determined by the doctor for each individual, with appropriate adjustments made as needed.

Products that combine theophylline with other medications should be avoided, especially during pregnancy (see page 86). These preparations typically contain theophylline, ephedrine, and a sedative (such as phenobarbitol or hydroxyzine). Since you should take as few medications as possible when you are pregnant, it makes sense to use a product that contains theophylline alone, especially since theophylline offers most of the benefit in the combination products.

Theophylline does get into breast milk. It is still acceptable when breast-feeding but the mother should be on the alert for irritability in the infant. If this occurs, notify your doctor as a theophylline dosage adjustment or an alternative medication for managing your asthma may remedy the situation.

Adrenalin-like Bronchodilators. You need to understand that Adrenalin-like bronchodilators in both inhaled and oral form are not officially approved by the Food and Drug Administration for use during pregnancy. Thus, if your doctor recommends one of these medications, be sure that you discuss with him your need for the medication in view of any risk of side effects. Ultimately, you are relying on the clinical judgment of your doctor that one of these medications is necessary to keep your airways open.

As of this writing, experience has shown that inhaled bronchodilators are acceptable for use during pregnancy if necessary. A case could be made that metaproterenol (Metaprel or Alupent) is preferable to albuterol (Proventil or Ventolin) because albuterol is a newer agent. However, there have been no clear-cut reports of specific problems with albuterol during pregnancy. Inhaled bronchodilators are preferable to oral bronchodilators during pregnancy because the inhaled medication acts directly on the airways, with less absorption into the body. As always, the inhaler must not be overused.

Interestingly, terbutaline (Brethine or Bricanyl) in pill form has been used by obstetricians to prevent premature labor in the third trimester. Therefore, consideration can be given to using terbutaline as a back-up medication if theophylline alone in proper dosage proves unrewarding.

Cromolyn Sodium. There have been no studies performed in the United States that show that cromolyn sodium (Intal) is safe for use during pregnancy. As a general rule, most pregnant asthma patients in this country are managed with a product that contains theophylline. However, there has been no pattern of birth defects noted to date in patients in other countries who have continued using cromolyn during pregnancy. Therefore, you are relying on your doctor's judgment if cromolyn is continued during pregnancy. You must understand that this decision is not without risk, although on the basis of limited experience with its use during pregnancy to date, it appears that the risk is quite small. Above all, you should become involved with the decision concerning use of medication during pregnancy.

Steroids. As you might expect, the use of steroids during pregnancy is always of great concern for both the mother and the baby. Doctors hesitate to use steroids because of the fear of congenital abnormalities in the fetus, especially cleft palate. On the other hand, untreated asthma that can lead to a drop in the mother's blood oxygen also carries a risk for the fetus. Therefore, when recent studies suggested that the risk of side effects and congenital abnormalities was not increased in infants of women taking the steroid prednisone (with an average dose of 8 milligrams daily), some of the concern for the use of this important medication during pregnancy was alleviated.

Pregnant women who use steroids should follow the guidelines for steroid use presented in Chapter 3. Steroids should be the last alternative for routine use. Theophylline and the Adrenalin-like bronchodilators should be used as optimally as possible in hope of avoiding the need for steroids. However, if steroids are needed, they should be used in as ideal a manner as possible (see page 110), preferably in inhaled form or on an alternate day, early morning basis.

For acute flares of asthma that are severe, it is better to control the symptoms with short-term use of steroids, if theophylline and the Adrenalin-like bronchodilators have proved unrewarding, than to let asthma symptoms linger. The decision to use steroids during pregnancy is a difficult decision for your doctor, but it is often better to err on the side of controlling difficult-to-manage asthma symptoms.

To date, no harmful effects to the fetus have been clearly shown to occur with the use of the inhaled steroid beclomethasone (Vanceril). As inhaled steroids act directly on the airways with little absorption into the rest of the body, it is preferable to use inhaled steroids rather than oral steroids whenever possible.

Nasal congestion is common during pregnancy and treatment is often unnecessary. However, for some women, the nasal congestion is so severe that they have troubled breathing through the nose and falling asleep. If this is the case, the choices for treatment include antihistamines with or without decongestants (see next section) and topical nasal steroids. With the availability of the topical nasal steroids, the need for oral steroids to treat nasal congestion during pregnancy is unusual. Products such as beclomethasone (Vancenase and Beconase) and flunisolide (Nasalide) are preferable to dexamethasone (Decadron Nasal Turbinaire) during pregnancy, as there is less absorption of the steroid into the body with the former products. However, the use of dexamethasone can be considered if beclomethasone and flunisolide have been insufficient to control the problem.

When an inhaled nasal steroid is used, it should be continued until the problem is brought under control. At that point, consideration can be given to the use of other medications such as a low dose of an antihistamine. Needless to say, all decisions in this regard should be discussed with your doctor. You should understand that there is a small potential risk with the use of any medication during pregnancy. You should discuss your thoughts with your doctor before using any of the inhaled steroid nasal preparations.

Antihistamines and Decongestants. Antihistamines and decongestants, like all other medications, are best avoided during pregnancy. If there is no alternative and if such a medication is absolutely necessary, it is best to use a product that is well known to your doctor and then to use it as sparingly as possible.

If nasal congestion needs to be treated, it is preferable to use an antihistamine in its short-acting form such as chlorpheniramine (Chlor-Trimeton). If chlorpheniramine makes you too sleepy or does not effectively control your nasal symptoms, alternatives which are thought to be acceptable during pregnancy include tripelennamine (Pyribenzamine), pheniramine, and diphenhydramine (Benadryl). Diphenhydramine is best reserved for the treatment of hives or allergic reactions. Hydroxyzine (Atarax and Vistaril) and cyproheptadine (Periactin), which are often used to treat hives, should be avoided during pregnancy. Brompheniramine (Bromfed or Dimetapp) are best avoided as there is a question of its risk during pregnancy.

Over-the-counter nasal decongestant sprays, such as Afrin, Neosynephrine, 4-Way, and Dristan, should be avoided during pregnancy. Although these products will initially decrease your nasal congestion, continued use can actually lead to increased nasal congestion. This is called rebound nasal congestion (rhinitis medicamentosa). Furthermore, continued use leads to difficulty in giving up the product. Don't be misled into thinking that you will use such a product sparingly. If you currently use one of these inhaled nasal sprays, discuss alternative medications with your doctor.

Oral decongestants such as pseudoephedrine (Sudafed, Afrinol, and Novafed), phenylpropanolamine (Propagest and Entex), and phenylephrine should be used only with your doctor's advice, as there are no studies that clearly indicate their safety during pregnancy. The addition of an oral decongestant is sometimes necessary, since an antihistamine used alone simply relieves nasal runniness and may not help the congestion. At this point, the choice of medications is simply a matter of judgment on your doctor's part in view of your particular situation.

Expectorants. Expectorants help you to clear your airways by coughing up secretions. Although in principle this makes sense, the usefulness of expectorants in asthma treatment is questionable with the products now available. Thus, expectorants should be avoided during pregnancy. Iodides specifically should be avoided because they could cause a goiter in the fetus, which could block the infant's airway and be life threatening. Theophylline combination products that contain iodide (such as Quadrinal) are best avoided.

Antibiotics. Certain antibiotics can be used during pregnancy for treatment of bacterial infections. Penicillin and its derivatives such as ampicillin are acceptable for use during pregnancy. If you are allergic to penicillin, erythromycin can be used with your obstetrician's approval. Tetracycline must be avoided during pregnancy due to concern for its possible effect on the infant's bone development and discoloration or staining of the infant's teeth. For the asthma patient, early treatment of an infection can sometimes reduce the risk of the infection triggering asthma symptoms. If you have any change in the color of mucus from your nose or chest (to yellow or green, in particular), fever, or pressure over your sinus areas, you should notify your doctor.

Allergy Injections. Allergy injections can be continued during pregnancy. A recent study failed to show any increase in congenital or maternal abnormalities when allergy shots were continued during pregnancy. For patients already on allergy shots, the dose and concentration should not be increased. The reason for this suggestion is that when the dose is being gradually elevated, as is the case when someone is just starting allergy shots, the risk of anaphylaxis (a generalized serious allergic reaction following an allergy shot) is slightly greater. Contraction of the uterus could occur with anaphylaxis, thereby triggering a miscarriage. Therefore, it is preferable not to begin allergy shots during pregnancy, as the dose has to be increased to note any improvement from the shots.

If allergy shots have improved your allergy or asthma symptoms, you can consider continuing shots while you are pregnant. Certainly it is important to notify your allergist as soon as you find out or suspect that you are pregnant, and to schedule an appointment to discuss whether you should continue allergy shots. Your allergist will review the benefits and risks of continuing allergy shots as well as the risk of stopping the shots. If you have found that your allergy shots have reduced your need for medication and that you have far less asthma symptoms since starting the shots, consideration should be given to continuing the shots throughout your pregnancy.

Medications to Avoid During Pregnancy. Table 9-1 lists those medications that should be avoided during pregnancy. These include tetracycline, iodides, aspirin and aspirin-containing products (as well as the cross-reacting medications, see page 34) in aspirin-sensitive individuals, and also the antihistamines hydroxyzine, cyproheptadine, and brompheniramine. All other medications, including over-the-counter medications, should be reviewed with your obstetrician and asthma doctor before you start to take them.

The treatment of asthma during pregnancy is very much the same as treatment of the nonpregnant patient who has asthma. Clearly, one of the problems is that there are but a few guidelines for doctors in deciding which medications are

---

**Medications Sometimes Used for Treating Asthma
That Should Be Avoided During Pregnancy**

* Tetracycline—can cause permanent staining of child's teeth

* Iodine (found in some asthma medications and often used as an expectorant)—can cause goiters in the infant

* Hydroxyzine (Atarax and Vistaril)

* Aspirin and tartrazine (yellow food dye #5)—should be avoided by individuals sensitive to these products

---

Table 9–1

acceptable for use during pregnancy. The information available in this area will no doubt expand in years to come. In the interim, it is wise to follow your doctor's suggestions closely and to use well-characterized medications that have been available for several years. With attention to sound asthma care during pregnancy, the prognosis for the mother and child is good. The secret to success is a close working relationship with your doctor, so that asthma symptoms are treated early and any medication suggestions made by your asthma doctor are clearly understood by you and approved by your obstetrician.

SUMMARY: ASTHMA AND PREGNANCY

1. Asthma occurs during pregnancy in 0.4 to 1.3 percent of all pregnant women.

2. The effect of pregnancy on asthma is summarized by the "rule of one-third": asthma symptoms improve during pregnancy for one-third of the women with asthma, remain the same for one-third, and become worse for one-third. A similar pattern follows with subsequent pregnancies. Those women whose asthma becomes more difficult during pregnancy are usually those whose asthma was more difficult to manage before pregnancy.

3. Asthma that is well managed and free of complications has little effect on pregnancy, as there are no clear-cut consequences from asthma during pregnancy for either the mother or the fetus.

4. If asthma medications are necessary during pregnancy, they must be reviewed with your asthma doctor as well as with your obstetrician. You must weigh the benefit of keeping your asthma under control against the small risk of side effects from asthma medications during pregnancy. Fortunately, experience has shown that many of the asthma medications can be used with little risk during pregnancy, although a clear-cut scientific study is unavailable for most medications.

5. Several of the theophylline products, bronchodilating inhalers, and even steroids (if there is no alternative) can be used during pregnancy, when necessary, with little risk of side effect to the fetus. As there is little experience with its use in pregnancy, cromolyn sodium should be avoided during pregnancy unless there is no alternative. Each of the medications typically used in asthma management is reviewed in this chapter in light of their acceptability for use during pregnancy. All medication decisions should be approved by both your asthma doctor and your obstetrician.

6. Allergy injections can be continued during pregnancy if they have improved your allergy and asthma symptoms. However, the dose should not be increased during pregnancy. It is preferable not to begin a program of allergy shots while you are pregnant.

7. Medications that should be avoided during pregnancy are summarized in Table 9–1.

8. With attention to sound asthma care during pregnancy, the overall prognosis for the mother and fetus is good.

◇ 10 ◇

Occupational Asthma

In reviewing the factors that can trigger asthma symptoms, one of the most commonly overlooked areas is the work place. The connection between the work environment and asthma symptoms is complicated by delayed asthma reactions, which often occur several hours after exposure. An important clue in making this association is whether there is any improvement in asthma symptoms when the person is not at work, such as over the weekend and during vacation times. Even though years of working in the same occupation have never triggered an asthma response, an occupational exposure could account for asthma symptoms at any time.

Occupational Asthma Not Necessarily Due to Allergy. Occupational asthma is not always due to an allergic response. Irritant reactions, whereby the offending industrial product stimulates the irritant receptors in the back of the throat and triggers an asthma response, can also explain some occupational asthma episodes. In addition, there is a large group of occupational asthma reactions where the cause is not known, as this field is still in its infancy.

Allergic Individuals Are at Greater Risk. Individuals who have an allergic tendency are thought to be at greater risk of developing asthma due to occupational exposure than are nonallergic individuals, regardless of whether the industrial agent is an allergen or an irritant. Nonallergic individuals can also develop occupational asthma but seem to develop symptoms only after a long period of exposure at work.

Asthma Flares Can Occur on a Delayed Basis. An asthma attack from an occupational exposure differs little from an asthma attack from any other cause. Asthma symptoms can occur within minutes of exposure, and an inhaled bronchodilator often is of benefit in this setting. However, for the delayed asthma response (which usually occurs four to six hours after exposure), the inhaled bronchodilators provide little relief. It is thought that delayed reactions are due to inflammation of the airway as opposed to muscle constriction of the airway. Although they are not blocked by inhaled bronchodilators and theophylline, the delayed reactions are blocked with the use of steroids. Steroids do not, however, block any immediate wheezing that occurs with exposure. Interestingly, cromolyn sodium (Intal) blocks both the immediate and the delayed reaction to an occupational allergen or irritant.

Your Occupational and Environmental History Is Essential. There is no readily available, clear-cut test that can definitely determine whether an occupational exposure is the cause of an asthma flare. It is therefore important to piece together all relevant information that can help your doctor make the correct diagnosis. A carefully taken medical history is essential, as direct contact with the offending agent need not occur. For example, cases have been reported where grain dust carried by the wind from nearby mills has triggered asthma symptoms. Consideration should be given to the possibility of exposure to irritants from industry near your home and work place. You should also tell your doctor if you have any hobbies that utilize chemicals, such as gardening, photography, or painting, as these may also contribute to asthma symptoms. As with other types of asthma, symptoms of occupational asthma can be as subtle as a cough. Other symptoms often associated with occupational asthma can mimic allergies, such as itchy red eyes (conjunctivitis), a sore throat, or a runny nose.

There Are Few Clear-Cut Tests for the Offending Agents. At times, allergy skin tests or blood tests (called RAST tests) can be helpful, but there is often no routine test available for a particular allergen or irritant. However, several occupational allergens have been identified and are available for testing at selected allergy centers in the United States.

Monitor Your Breathing Tests. As with any type of asthma, a person who has occupational asthma can have a normal breathing test (spirometry) result. However, when the person is having asthma symptoms, spirometry should reveal a drop in lung function. If the patient's breathing test improves after an inhaled bronchodilator is used, this indicates that the patient has asthma. If the symptoms are due to a delayed asthma reaction, there is usually little improvement from a bronchodilator; in this setting, a short course of steroids is often given to improve symptoms, and the breathing test is repeated on a different day. If the occupational exposure has gone on for a lengthy time period, such as several years, it is possible that the airway blockage can become fixed and therefore be irreversible. It is important to identify occupational asthma early so that your doctor can periodically repeat your breathing test and offer appropriate suggestions.

Challenging Your Airways with the Potential Occupational Agent. One way of determining whether an occupational agent is causing asthma symptoms is to actually inhale the agent and then to monitor your breathing test over several hours. This is called a bronchial provocation test. This test is not without risk, as a dramatic drop in the functioning of the airways can occur in some individuals. Therefore, this test should be performed by a specialist whose office or testing facility is set up to manage any possible emergencies that could result from the test.

Breathing Tests (Spirometry) May Be Lower in Cigarette Smokers. Cigarette smoking complicates proper assessment of occupational asthma, as cigarette smokers often have abnormal breathing tests. For example, tests of the smaller airways are often lower in cigarette smokers. Needless to say, the symptoms of occupational asthma can be made worse by cigarette smoking.

Occupations That Can Cause Asthma. Table 10-1 summarizes the agents and work settings that have been associated with occupational asthma. The problem can occur in heavy industry as well as in the supermarket. Examples include: (a) meat wrapper's asthma, caused by fumes from the breakdown of polyvinylchloride plastic (PVC) when heat is used to cut and seal the plastic during meat wrapping; (b) baker's asthma, caused by inhaling flour in a poorly ventilated work place, (c) cotton worker's asthma, called byssinosis or Monday illness, the cause of which is not fully understood; and (d) polyurethane workers's asthma, due to exposure to the chemical toluene diisocyanate (TDI).

Identifying and Avoiding the Offending Agent. Treatment of occupational asthma is frequently the same as treatment of asthma that is not related to an occupational exposure. Needless to say, the offending agent should be avoided if possible. Often this involves first documenting that the suspected agent is in fact the culprit. This can be a difficult and costly process for the industry. It is important for industries that have been shown to be potential risks to asthma sufferers to share this information with their present and prospective employees. When a chemical or dust has been identified as a potential offender, the industry should routinely monitor its facilities—for example, to check for leaks that might increase the exposure. There is no substitute for proper ventilation and efforts to contain exposure to accepted levels. Alternative measures such as face masks can also be beneficial but are uncomfortable to wear and often impair sight and breathing.

Changing Employment Can Be A Difficult Decision. A worker with occupational asthma may face the difficult decision of whether to continue to work in the same industry.

Some Causes of Occupational Asthma

Occupation	Material
Bakers, flour mill workers	Flour
Chemical and petroleum industry	Ammonia, hydrochloric acid, chlorine, sulfur dioxide
Detergent industry	Bacterial enzymes
Electrical trade	Soldering fluxes
Farmers	Organic phosphorus used in insecticides; animal dander
Grain handlers, grain elevator operators	Grain dust, insects, and mites
Hairdressers	Henna
Laboratory workers around animals	Animal dander and rat urine
Meat wrappers	Polyvinylchloride (PVC) by-products
Metal foundry workers	Formaldehyde
Metal platers	Salts of nickel
Metal refiners	Salts of platinum
Oil and food workers	Castor beans, green coffee beans, papain, pancreatic extracts
Pharmaceutical industry	Ampicillin, penicillin, piperazine
Plastic, resin, and rubber industries	By-products including phthalic anhydride, trimellitic anhydride, ethylene diamine
Polyurethane industry	Toluene diisocyanate (TDI)
Printers	Vegetable gums
Textile industry	Cotton dust, flax, hemp
Veterinarians	Animal dander and hair
Wood workers, sawmill operators, and carpenters	Wood dusts

Table 10–1

At times this becomes an economic decision, as seniority a worker has built up in an industry often is not transferable to another field. Efforts should be made by all industries to set up an equitable system to allow for job transfer in situations such as this. When a change of employment is not possible, you should consult with your asthma doctor to devise a program that utilizes preventative medications on a daily basis before exposure. Careful follow-up with your doctor, including routine breathing tests, is essential if the worker decides to remain in an industry that has triggered occupational asthma.

Asthma Medication Choices. The full range of asthma medications can be considered when treating occupational asthma. Cromolyn sodium (Intal) may be the best choice for some individuals, since it blocks both the immediate and the delayed asthma response to an occupational agent, and does not contain steroids. However, cromolyn used by itself may not be sufficient to control asthma symptoms for some people. Alternatives to the use of cromolyn include: (a) Theophylline—when used on a routine basis to keep the airways open, theophylline can block the immediate asthma response to an industrial agent, but cannot block the delayed asthma response. (b) Inhaled bronchodilators—when used prior to entering the work place, these will also block immediate but not delayed asthma symptoms. (c) Inhaled (when possible) or oral steroids—these block the delayed asthma response but not the immediate asthma response when exposed to an offending agent. The combination of theophylline or a bronchodilating inhaler along with steroids to block the delayed asthma reactions is often considered as an alternative or supplement to cromolyn. As is always the case, oral steroids are the last alternative, and should be reserved for use when theophylline and the Adrenalin-like bronchodilators prove unrewarding.

If There Is Risk of Irreversible Airway Blockage, It Is Best to Change Your Work Environment. To continue in the work place after it has been determined to be a factor leading to your asthma symptoms can carry great risk, even if appropriate preventative measures are followed (such as the use of preexposure medications). Asthma in this setting could eventually result in fixed airway obstruction—that is, chest symptoms and breathing tests that fail to respond to medication. Therefore, a person with occupational asthma should be certain that he is fully informed about the risks of continuing to work in the same environment. Given the information available today, the most appropriate choice for most individuals with clearly documented occupational asthma is a change of work environment.

SUMMARY: OCCUPATIONAL ASTHMA

1. Asthma can be triggered by exposure to offending agents in the work place. The possibility of occupational asthma should be considered in all asthma patients.

2. Occupational asthma can be caused by irritants as well as by allergens. Often no specific agent can be found to account for occupational asthma.

3. Allergic individuals seem to have a greater chance of developing asthma due to occupational exposure, although nonallergic individuals are also at risk after a long period of exposure.

4. Asthma flares can occur immediately on exposure to an offending agent or can occur on a delayed basis, several hours after exposure.

5. It is important to review whether the places in which you live and work, as well as surrounding areas, might be associated with industrial exposure. A helpful clue is the absence of symptoms when you are out of the environment in question, such as during weekends or vacations.

6. There are few clear-cut tests that can determine whether asthma is caused by an occupational exposure. Breathing tests should be performed routinely. Challenging your

airways with the potential offending agent (bronchial provocation testing) is sometimes considered, although this is not without risk.

7. Some occupations that are associated with a potential asthma risk are listed in Table 10–1.

8. The steps for treating occupational asthma are: (a) identify and avoid the offending agent; (b) change employment if advised to do so by your doctor; (c) use medications before exposure if avoidance is impossible, but only if you understand that there is a risk of serious, irreversible airway obstruction associated with long-term occupational asthma; and (d) consider the use of a face mask, knowing its limitations.

9. Theophylline and the bronchodilating inhalers are useful in blocking asthma reactions that are immediate, occurring within minutes of exposure to an occupational agent. Steroids block delayed reactions, which occur up to several hours after exposure. Cromolyn sodium (Intal) offers the advantage of blocking both immediate and delayed reactions. If theophylline or the bronchodilating inhalers prove ineffective initially, consideration can be given to trying cromolyn or adding steroids (preferably in the inhaled rather than the oral form).

10. Given the information available today, if occupational asthma has been clearly documented, it is best to change your work environment if at all possible.

◊ 11 ◊

Surgery and Anesthesia

All asthma patients who require surgery should be closely monitored by their asthma doctor as well as by the surgery team. Proper assessment of your asthma is important prior to surgery, as reorganization of your medication program may be required. If you have taken steroids during the past twelve months, a steroid "boost" (a large dose of steroids) prior to and after surgery is essential. Your asthma doctor should discuss with the anesthesiologist the choice of anesthesia and the appropriate medications to use if you experience any asthma flares during surgery. Therefore, if you are going to have elective (non-emergency) surgery, notify your asthma doctor well in advance so that he can confer with the surgeon and anesthesiologist.

Preoperative Preparation. As part of the preoperative evaluation, your lung function as measured by a breathing test (spirometry) is important, as this provides an objective measure of your breathing status. Although your chest may appear to be clear when your doctor listens with his stethoscope, your spirometry results could be dramatically different. For those individuals whose asthma is truly difficult to manage, the amount of oxygen in the arterial blood should be checked. This is called an arterial blood gas determina-

240

tion. If you have been taking steroids on a regular basis and have noticed that bruises and cuts seem to heal slowly, this should be discussed with your doctor beforehand in the case of elective surgery. Just prior to surgery, your doctor will carefully check for any sign of infection by ordering a complete blood count and a sedimentation rate. A repeat of your chest X-ray examination is standard procedure if you will be having general anesthesia.

Choice of Anesthesia. An important decision for the asthma patient having surgery is the type of anesthesia to be used. Be certain that you take part in any decision regarding the choice between local or general anesthesia, although often the nature of the surgery will determine that there is no choice.

Local Anesthesia. Local anesthesia refers to medications injected directly into the surgical area or the nerves that supply the area. Local anesthetics such as lidocaine (Xylocaine) are typically injected just under the skin to provide numbing of the site of the operation. When a local anesthetic is injected more deeply below the skin into the nerves that control the surgical area, this is called a nerve block. Nerve blocks are often used when operating on the arms or legs or when delivering a baby in order to numb the birth canal. When local anesthetics are placed in the spinal canal, this is called spinal anesthesia. This form of anesthesia is used for abdominal surgery or surgery on the legs. When the local anesthetic is placed just above the lining of the spinal canal, this is called an epidural. As local anesthesia does not usually affect the patient's breathing, it is often a good choice for patients with asthma.

General Anesthesia. The term general anesthesia means that you lose consciousness in a controlled setting. In most cases, the anesthetic agent is a gas inhaled through a mask. A breathing tube is placed in your airway once you are "asleep" to be certain that the anesthesiologist has control of your airways. A breathing tube is used for most patients who have general anesthesia, especially when the surgery is extensive. There is always a risk of complications with general anesthesia, regardless of whether you have asthma, but it is a small risk, especially if prior to surgery your breathing status is properly assessed and any necessary medications are given. Although local anesthesia is usually preferable for a person with asthma, general anesthesia does offer the advantage that the anesthesiologist has control of the patient's airways with the breathing tube. In addition, most of the anesthetics used today during surgery on asthma patients (such as halothane) offer the advantage of relaxing the muscles surrounding the air tubes, thereby reducing the likelihood of triggering asthma symptoms.

Asthma Medications for the Surgical Patient

Theophylline. Your medication requirements must be reassessed prior to surgery. For patients who require theophylline on a daily basis and will be having general anesthesia, most physicians choose to administer theophylline during surgery in the form of intravenous Aminophylline. This offers the anesthesiologist and the surgeon the advantage of greater control of the patient's blood theophylline level. Thus, if you experience any change in heart rate during surgery that might possibly be linked to theophylline, the intravenous flow of theophylline going into your body can easily and quickly be stopped. However, if you took an oral dose of long-acting theophylline before surgery, it would be impossible to control your theophylline level. During surgery, the intravenous theophylline dose is usually administered in conservative doses, such as 0.5 milligrams per kilogram of body weight per hour. Needless to say, this replaces any oral dose of theophylline you normally take.

Adrenalin-like Bronchodilators. The oral Adrenalin-like medications such as metaproterenol (Metaprel or Alupent), albuterol (Ventolin or Proventil), or terbutaline (Bricanyl or Brethine) are usually discontinued prior to surgery, as they may cause a rapid heart rate. In their place, inhaled medications such as metaproterenol or isoetharine (Bronkosol) can be administered with a nebulizer. The use of a nebulizer offers the advantage of directing the medication to the airways with less stimulation of the heart. Although inhalers such as albuterol (Ventolin or Proventil), terbutaline (Brethaire), or metaproterenol (Metaprel or Alupent) can be continued during the preoperative period, they are often replaced by medications used with a nebulizer, since the nebulized breathing treatment is of longer duration and not as dependent on proper technique for a successful result.

Steroids. The body's normal response to physical stress such as surgery is to release greater amounts of steroids than are normally present in the blood. These additional steroids help the body handle the stress more effectively. If you take steroids on a regular basis, your body does not release additional steroids during times of stress as it normally would. For this reason supplemental steroids are required both before and after surgery if you have taken steroids during the previous twelve months. Steroids are usually given at the higher dose beginning the day before surgery and continuing through the day after surgery. Steroid doses during this time period can range from 30 to 125 milligrams, taken intravenously as frequently as every 6 hours. It is usually possible during the second postoperative day to discontinue the additional steroids and return to your normal steroid dose. As is the case with routine steroid use, steroid doses related to surgery must be determined on an individual basis.

Medications That Should Be Avoided. Medications that should be avoided while in the hospital include aspirin, products that contain aspirin, nonsteroid anti-inflammatory medications (such as ibuprofen and naproxen—see Table 2–4), indomethacin, phenylbutazone, and tartrazine (yellow food dye #5). You may want to ask the nurses to place these precautions on the front of your hospital chart so that they are not overlooked. You should also ask your asthma doctor to review any medications the surgery staff will be prescribing for you.

The Day of Surgery. With these steps completed during the preoperative time period, your surgery should proceed smoothly. By the day of surgery, your intravenous medications have already been ordered and timed so that they coincide with the proposed time of surgery. A good choice for preoperative sedation is hydroxyzine (Atarax or Vistaril), since it tends not to suppress your breathing. At that point, there is little to do except stay calm and be confident that all details have been attended to.

Postoperative Care. The postoperative period is as important as the preoperative period, and your breathing status must be followed carefully. Deep breathing using a device called an incentive spirometer encourages you to clear secretions in your chest. This is important in order to avoid small areas of your lungs from closing due to the build-up of secretions, a process called atelectasis. The use of inhaled bronchodilators should be continued during the postoperative period. Intravenous theophylline can be discontinued and replaced by your oral theophylline preparation once you begin eating again. The decision of how long to continue taking additional steroids is made on an individual basis, although it is usually possible during the second postoperative day to return to your normal dose.

Emergency Surgery. If surgery is required on an emergency basis, provisions should be made to guard against complications with your asthma by following the guidelines discussed above to the greatest extent possible. If you use steroids on a regular basis or have taken steroids during the past year, it is essential that you carry this information with you in the form of a card or a Medi-Alert bracelet, since you would require supplemental steroids in the event of an accident or emergency surgery. Your asthma doctor should be contacted if possible during a medical emergency.

SUMMARY: SURGERY AND ANESTHESIA

1. When an asthma patient requires surgery, coordination is necessary among the surgeon, the anesthesiologist, and the doctor caring for your asthma.

2. Your breathing status must be checked just prior to surgery, using an objective measure such as spirometry. You should also be examined for any signs of infection. A chest X-ray should be performed if you are having general anesthesia.

3. Local anesthesia, which simply numbs the surgical area, is always preferable to general anesthesia.

4. Your asthma does not necessarily present a risk during general anesthesia as long as your breathing status is acceptable when going into surgery. During surgery, the anesthesiologist has control of your breathing through the use of a breathing tube placed in your airway.

5. If you are having local anesthesia, your normal dose of oral theophylline may not need to be adjusted. With general anesthesia, the oral dose of theophylline is discontinued and replaced with intravenous theophylline (Aminophylline) to allow control of the theophylline dose during surgery.

6. Adrenalin-like bronchodilators that are taken by mouth should usually be discontinued before general anesthesia, as they can increase the heart rate. The best means of using these medications prior to surgery is with a nebulizer, although inhalers can also be used.

7. If you have taken steroids during the last twelve months, supplemental steroids should be given both before and after surgery. Steroid doses are determined by your doctor on an individual basis. Supplemental steroids are especially important during this period for asthma patients who take steroids on a regular basis.

8. Medications that should be avoided while in the hospital include aspirin and products that contain aspirin, as well as medications that cross-react with aspirin (see Tables 2–3 and 2–4). These precautions should be written on the front of your hospital chart.

9. The use of steroids, intravenous theophylline, and the inhaled bronchodilators should be continued during the postoperative period. Once you are eating again, your normal dose of oral theophylline can replace the intravenous theophylline. It is usually possible during the second postoperative day to discontinue the additional steroids and return to your normal steroid dose.

10. If you use steroids on a regular basis or have taken steroids during the past year, you should carry this information with you in the form of a card or Medi-Alert bracelet, since you would require supplemental steroids in the event of an accident or emergency surgery.

◇ 12 ◇

Psychological Aspects

Asthma Is Not a Psychosomatic Illness. By far the most widespread myth concerning asthma is that it is a psychosomatic illness and that the problem is "all in the head." This is not true, and it is important for family, friends, acquaintances, and employers, as well as for the asthma patient himself, to know that this is not true. Although emotional upset can trigger or aggravate asthma, one must first have the underlying physical problem in order to have asthma symptoms.

Emotional Support of the Asthma Sufferer. It is wrong to view someone with asthma as emotionally disturbed, but it is equally wrong to ignore underlying psychological, behavioral, or emotional problems which may be related to asthma. There is no question that asthma that is chronic and difficult to manage can have a negative impact on one's personal relationships and family life as well as on one's self-image. Often by simply discussing your feelings about asthma with your doctor, you will realize that they are normal feelings and find a sense of relief. If counseling is recommended, this should be viewed as a positive suggestion that can help you help yourself, as opposed to a sign of failure. There is no rule that says that you must be able to cope with your problems by yourself at all times. If you need assistance, you should not deny yourself the opportunity of talking with someone, as this can at times make a big difference in the direction of your asthma care.

Alternative Psychological Approaches. Beyond emotional support from your asthma doctor, family, and friends, other psychologically oriented approaches to asthma care include relaxation techniques (such as biofeedback), hypnosis, family counseling, psychotherapy, and psychoanalysis. Each has its place, and the decision as to which approach is best for you should be discussed with the specialist to whom you have been referred. This provides an opportunity for you to voice your opinions about the approach you ultimately will take to best handle this aspect of your care, and also allows you the chance to be certain that you feel comfortable with your psychologist or psychiatrist.

Biofeedback. Biofeedback has received a great deal of attention as a method of teaching asthma patients to relax so that bronchodilation (opening of the airways) can occur. The usefulness of this approach has not yet been fully confirmed but it holds promise for some asthma patients. Biofeedback involves setting up a "feedback loop." Wiring attached to the skin or muscles sends information (such as temperature change in the skin) to an electronic sensor, which is displayed to the patient. The effect of various stimuli, such as reading about asthma or talking about family relationships, are "fed back" to the patient so that he or she can see firsthand the impact these topics have on his state of relaxation. With training, the person learns to distinguish tension from relaxation and to adjust to the feeling of tension and favor relaxation. Ultimately, the asthma patient learns to relax and to voluntarily control, to some extent, the temperature of his skin, as well as hopefully to bring about relaxation of the muscles which control the tone of the airways. As there is little risk associated with biofeedback, it may well be worth a try if suggested by your doctor.

Hypnosis. The role of hypnosis in asthma is still quite controversial and reports vary as to its success. Hypnosis should not be viewed as a potential cure for asthma but rather as an adjunct to comprehensive care for some individuals. With hypnosis, the asthma patient utilizes breathing exercises or other hypnotic suggestions to bring about relaxation. Routine self-hypnosis can be utilized as an additional approach to asthma management for some people. Needless to say, hypnosis should be directed by someone skilled in the technique and by someone who is also prepared to support you through any problems that may arise.

Family Counseling. When asthma emergencies and symptoms occur frequently, and when the cost of asthma care and medications sometimes consume as much as 10 to 20 percent of a family's income, it is not surprising that the impact of asthma can extend to the entire family. Often there is a sense of frustration and hidden resentment by other family members that may well be normal, but that should nonetheless be addressed with professional counseling. Asthma often places great strain on working parents when they must take care of a child with asthma as well as meet the demands of their family and their jobs. If a child's frequent asthma symptoms interfere with the family's recreation and leisure time as well as with his daily routine, the child may try to hide his asthma symptoms, even if this is impossible. Any of these factors may or may not play a role in your situation. Certainly family counseling, which at times is done in the house, may be worthwhile for some families.

One approach used in family counseling is to have the entire family become more aware of the factors that precipitate asthma symptoms as well as the appropriate medications, so that it becomes a family project to help control asthma symptoms. Another approach is to examine family interactions that may have impact on the child with asthma. Separation of a child from his parents and family (''parentectomy'') formerly was recommended to remove the child with asthma from an emotionally unstable environment. This approach, which has fallen into disfavor, is not thought to be as beneficial as family therapy, which retains the normal composition of the family unit.

Psychotherapy. Psychotherapy is directed toward a more thorough understanding of your emotional state and should be conducted by a trained professional (either a psychiatric social worker, clinical psychologist or psychiatrist). One of the goals of therapy is to give you a greater understanding of any problems or personality traits that may contribute to your asthma symptoms. Because of the cost involved in this approach as well as the time commitment (which may involve years), ask your asthma doctor for a referral to a specialist who has expertise in working with asthma patients.

Confidence Associated with Asthma Self-Management. You should take advantage of educational seminars on asthma to enhance your understanding of your condition so that you feel that it is under better control. It is my belief that if you have a written program that summarizes exactly what you are to do if asthma symptoms flare, you will have a sense of confidence that your asthma symptoms can be managed. This method also tends to reduce stress at a time when you should try to relax. This is one way of reducing the fear often associated with wheezing and difficulty catching your breath.

Ignoring Symptoms or Neglecting to Take Medications Is a Serious Problem. If you tend to ignore your asthma symptoms or to feel helpless when asthma symptoms flare, you should share these concerns with your doctor. It is important not to give up, or to feel that there is nothing that you can do to have better control of your asthma. As a first step, be sure to follow your medication program closely. If your back-up medication is not working, see your doctor early before your symptoms become worse. You should never ignore asthma symptoms, hoping that they will go away on their own. If you have developed a pattern of ignoring your asthma symptoms, it may help to have a psychiatrist on your team to work with you and your doctor.

Although asthma is not a psychosomatic illness, emotional

upset can clearly be a factor that worsens asthma symptoms. An approach to asthma management should not ignore the patient's emotional state, as it can clearly have impact on the long-term outcome for the asthma patient. Think of yourself not as an asthmatic, but as a person who has asthma—this distinction will ensure that all aspects of your condition will be considered, not merely the physical manifestations of asthma.

SUMMARY: PSYCHOLOGICAL ASPECTS

1. The myth that asthma is a psychosomatic illness has been a tremendous burden for the asthma patient. However, it is true that asthma can be made worse by emotional upset.

2. If emotional upset does contribute to your asthma symptoms, psychological counseling may be necessary to supplement your asthma care.

3. The roles of various psychologically oriented approaches to asthma care are discussed, including biofeedback, hypnosis, family counseling, educational seminars, and psychotherapy.

4. If you tend to ignore your asthma symptoms or neglect to take your medications as directed, these issues should be brought to your doctor's attention.

5. Think of yourself not as an asthmatic but as a person who has asthma.

PART FOUR

◇◇◇◇◇

Asthma out of Control

◇ 13 ◇

Status Asthmaticus

Status asthmaticus is the medical term used to describe severe asthma symptoms that fail to respond to routine treatment. This is a serious, potentially life-threatening condition that requires hospitalization and intensive medical management.

What Happens in the Airways During Status Asthmaticus. When asthma is out of control during status asthmaticus, there is increased constriction of the airways, increased inflammation within the lining of the airways, and increased mucus plugging the airways. As the airways become more and more obstructed, it becomes increasingly difficult for the asthma patient to breathe.

To compensate for the blockage within the airways, the normal response of the body is an increase in the rate of breathing (hyperventilation). The initial result of hyperventilation is that the amount of oxygen in the blood is maintained or increases while the carbon dioxide level in the blood decreases. However, if the blockage in the airways is severe or if the patient becomes fatigued from the effort of breathing, the oxygen level eventually decreases and, more seriously, the carbon dioxide level increases because it cannot be effectively exhaled. Therefore, if the carbon dioxide level in the blood approaches or exceeds the normal level during an acute asthma flare with rapid breathing, this is a serious sign, indicating dangerous obstruction of the airways.

In order to monitor the oxygen and carbon dioxide levels in the blood, a sample of blood is taken from an artery, usually in the arm. If the carbon dioxide level of this blood is elevated and does not decrease with intensive medication management, a breathing tube may have to be inserted into the airway to support the patient's breathing with a ventilator (a machine which helps the patient to breathe). Without mechanical ventilation, abnormalities in the oxygen and carbon dioxide levels in the blood can result in irregular heartbeats, which could be fatal. However, with close monitoring of asthma patients during status asthmaticus, death from asthma is usually preventable.

Typical Patient History. The usual patient history for status asthmaticus reveals wheezing that has been ignored for several days in the hope that it would pass. Often, asthma symptoms were triggered by an upper respiratory infection, medications were taken haphazardly, and the doctor caring for the patient's asthma was not contacted early enough. Status asthmaticus also occurs in a small group of patients whose asthma comes on so suddenly and is so severe that medications available to the patient at home are not sufficient. Asthma flares that begin suddenly can also be caused by sulfites (page 47), or products that contain aspirin or cross-react with aspirin (page 33). In contrast to adults, infants and young children can develop severe asthma symptoms quite rapidly, especially in association with an upper airway infection such as a cold.

Wheezing May Be Absent. If wheezing is not heard on examination of the chest during a severe asthma flare, this is a poor sign suggesting that there is not enough air movement in and out of the airways to produce a wheezing sound. Wheezing and coughing are usually present during status asthmaticus, along with a rapid heart rate and sweating. The patient uses all his chest muscles to breathe and the rate of breathing is rapid.

Diagnostic Tests. Breathing tests (spirometry) provide an objective measurement of the extent of the airway blockage, and should be compared with breathing tests that were performed when the patient was free of asthma symptoms. During status asthmaticus, the breathing test results are typically quite low and improve only slightly with bronchodilating medications. A chest X-ray is usually taken to rule out the possibility of any of the complications of asthma, such as collapse of the lung resulting from air in the chest cavity (pneumothorax) or any signs of infection. An arterial blood gas test is used to check the oxygen and carbon dioxide levels in the arterial blood. This test is a measure of how well you are breathing. As discussed above, if the oxygen in the blood decreases and the carbon dioxide (the body's waste product) increases, mechanical support for your breathing may be necessary.

Treatment of Status Asthmaticus. Asthma symptoms that fail to respond to inhaled bronchodilators, injected Adrenalin, or intravenous theophylline fit the description of status asthmaticus. As a first step in treatment of status asthmaticus, your doctor will try to understand the factors that triggered your asthma symptoms (such as an infection, or a medication such as aspirin), to know your present regimen of medications and when you last took them, and to be informed if you have any other medical problems such as thyroid or heart trouble.

General Measures. Often while your doctor is talking with you, arrangements are being made for you to have an Adrenalin injection or an inhalation treatment using a bronchodilator such as metaproterenol or isoetharine. Oxygen is usually given, which increases the oxygen that enters your airways and also helps to relax the airways somewhat. A needle is placed into a vein in your hand or forearm in order to provide fluids; this is called an intravenous line. Fluids are an important part of asthma therapy as they help to liquefy secretions, especially during status asthmaticus when patients tend to be somewhat dehydrated. In addition, the intravenous line is used to administer medications rapidly and directly into the bloodstream.

Sedatives Must Be Avoided During Status Asthmaticus, Except When the Patient's Breathing Is Being Controlled by Mechanical Ventilation. It may seem logical to give a patient who is having difficulty breathing a medication to help him calm down and rest. However, with rare exception, *IT IS A SERIOUS MISTAKE TO GIVE SLEEPING PILLS OR SEDATIVES TO ANY ASTHMA PATIENT WHO IS HAVING DIFFICULTY BREATHING.* Sedatives suppress the patient's respiratory rate and possibly his urge to breathe, which is exactly the opposite of what is necessary to avoid respiratory collapse and mechanical ventilation.

Medications Used During Status Asthmaticus. The same medications that have been described for routine asthma management are used for patients during status asthmaticus, except that they are used more intensively. Theophylline is administered intravenously, inhaled bronchodilators are administered via a nebulizer at two-hour intervals initially, and steroids are given intravenously in large doses at four- to six-hour intervals. A description of the use of each of the medication groups during status asthmaticus is presented below (see also Chapter 3).

Adrenalin and Adrenalin-like Medications. In the emergency room, epinephrine (Adrenalin) is still the most common first-line approach to asthma that is out of control. Adrenalin by injection is given two or three times if necessary, with twenty minutes between injections. The usual dose for adults is 0.2 to 0.3 milliliters of Adrenalin (1:1000 concentration) given just under the skin (subcutaneously). If there is little improvement after the third dose, Adrenalin should not be administered again, out of concern for causing irregular heartbeats. You should inform the emergency room doctor if you have a history of high blood pressure, thyroid problems, or heart problems, which may indicate that inhaled medications would be a better choice for you than Adrenalin.

Terbutaline by Injection. Injected terbutaline (Brethine or Bricanyl) can be used in place of Adrenalin. In theory, terbutaline offers the advantage of acting more directly on the lungs with less effect on the heart than Adrenalin, although in practice this distinction is not as clear-cut. If there is any question as to the condition of the patient's heart, the use of inhaled bronchodilators in place of injected terbutaline or Adrenalin should be considered.

Inhaled Bronchodilators Administered with a Neb-ulizer Can Be Used in Place of Adrenalin. Inhaled bronchodilators such as metaproterenol (Alupent or Meta-prel) or isoetharine (Bronkosol) administered with a nebulizer are appropriate for use in place of Adrenalin. The advantage of inhaled bronchodilators is that they act directly on the lungs with less effect on the heart and they do not cause as much shakiness and pallor as Adrenalin. Inhaled bronchodilators can be given as frequently as every two hours in the early stages of status asthmaticus, as long as the pulse rate does not increase greatly (over 130 beats per minute). When there is improvement in the patient's breathing status, the inhaled bronchodilator treatments are given at four- to six-hour intervals.

Intermittent Positive Pressure Breathing Should Be Avoided. IPPB machines deliver bronchodilating medications under pressure, with the idea that the medication will then be better able to penetrate into the lungs. However, there is no evidence to date that shows that an IPPB machine is any more effective in delivering the medication than a nebulizer. As a matter of fact, some physicians believe that a nebulizer allows for better distribution of the medication because the medication is taken in with slow deep breaths. The major concern with IPPB machines is that the additional pressure they generate could cause injury to the lungs. In view of these factors, the IPPB machine is best avoided in favor of using a nebulizer.

Alupent Unit Dosing Packets Are Free of Sulfites. Patients who are sensitive to sulfites need to know that Alupent unit dosing packets are the only inhaled bronchodilating solution currently available that does not contain sulfites. Both terbutaline and metaproterenol in multidose containers contain sulfites as preservatives.

Isoproterenol Can Be Given Intravenously To Certain Critical Patients. Isoproterenol given intravenously is reserved for patients who have failed to respond to intensive medical therapy, and for whom respiratory failure seems imminent or for whom mechanical ventilation has already been necessary. Careful observation in a hospital intensive care unit is necessary if isoproterenol is given intravenously, as it does have the potential of triggering irregular heartbeats. Intravenous isoproterenol is used along with other asthma medications such as intravenous Aminophylline, and can be discontinued as soon as the patient's condition begins to improve. It is preferable not to use this medication for patients with any heart or blood pressure problems. Most doctors who use isoproterenol intravenously limit its use primarily to children.

Theophylline. The only theophylline product available for use intravenously is Aminophylline. As with oral theophylline products (see page 78), the appropriate dose must be adjusted to ensure that the patient's blood theophylline level is within the therapeutic range (10 to 20 micrograms per milliliter of blood serum). The theophylline dose must be determined individually for each person, and the theophylline level checked periodically to be certain that it is within the ideal range. Typically, intravenous theophylline is given on a continuous basis as opposed to every few hours. Side effects of theophylline include jitteriness, headache, nausea, and vomiting. If you experience any of these side effects, mention this to your doctor. If you have heart or liver problems or if you are taking a medication that affects the body's metabolism of theophylline, be sure that your doctor is aware of this, as adjustments in your theophylline dose may have to be made. For a list of factors that affect the theophylline level, see Table 3–12.

Steroids. Inflammation and mucus within the airways is a major problem during status asthmaticus, and steroids are usually necessary to help clear the airways. The serious risks from steroids come only with long-term use. *THEREFORE, IT WOULD BE DANGEROUS TO WITHHOLD STEROIDS DURING STATUS ASTHMATICUS FOR FEAR OF STEROID DEPENDENCY OR STEROID SIDE EFFECTS.* Intravenous steroids require from four to six hours to work, so they should be administered as soon as possible during status asthmaticus.

Steroid Dose for Status Asthmaticus. The dose of steroid used to treat status asthmaticus varies among doctors. Most would agree that steroids should be administered in sufficiently high dose to bring asthma symptoms under control. Steroid doses range from 100 to 200 milligrams for hydrocortisone (Solu-Cortef), and from 40 to 125 milligrams for methylprednisolone (Solu-Medrol), every four to six hours per day until asthma symptoms are under better control. Some physicians recommend even higher doses of steroids (up to one gram of Solu-Medrol) for a short time, until asthma symptoms are under control. Although somewhat controversial, higher doses of steroid appear to date to be acceptable for short-term use.

Timing of Steroids During Status Asthmaticus. Close monitoring of the patient's progress during status asthmaticus determines if the steroid dose can be decreased. Often the dose is kept the same but the time interval between doses is increased. Unlike steroids taken on a regular basis, steroids used during status asthmaticus are not administered as a single morning dose, since more intensive medication therapy is necessary. However, as the patient's condition begins to improve, consideration can be given to administering steroids only once a day, in the morning, as one of the final steps in tapering the steroid dose.

Steroids Can Cause Changes in Potassium and Blood Sugar, Which Should Be Monitored. A check of the patient's potassium level (which may be lower than normal) and blood sugar level (which may be increased) is important for patients who are taking steroids. Alterations in the potassium and blood sugar levels are easily corrected and are not a reason to discontinue the use of steroids during status asthmaticus.

Antibiotics. As previously mentioned, viral illnesses (which do not respond to antibiotics) account for more asthma flares than do bacterial infections (which do respond to antibiotics). However, when asthma symptoms persist, mucus plugging the airways can become infected with bacteria. For this reason some physicians administer an antibiotic such as ampicillin, erythromycin, or one of the cephalosporins to clear up any potentially infected mucus during status asthmaticus.

Physical Therapy Such as Percussion and Postural Drainage Can Help Clear Mucus Plugs When Asthma Symptoms Have Been Longstanding. When asthma symptoms persist, mucus secretions can accumulate and eventually plug the airways. The patient should be encouraged to cough in order to clear mucus plugs, although this effort is often not successful. In addition, if mucus plugging is extensive, small areas of the lung might collapse—a condition called atelectasis. Mucus plugs can sometimes be dislodged by firmly tapping (percussing) specific areas of the back and chest while the patients sits or reclines in various positions. This technique is called percussion and postural drainage, and is typically performed in the hospital after the patient has been given an inhaled bronchodilator (see page 273).

Mechanical Ventilation. When the management approach outlined above proves unrewarding and the patient begins to tire, it may become necessary to place a tube in the patient's airway to allow a mechanical ventilator to take over the work of breathing. The doctor decides whether a patient requires mechanical ventilation on the basis of careful monitoring of the patient's arterial blood oxygen and carbon dioxide levels. The appearance and stamina of the patient are also factors in this decision.

Once the patient's breathing is controlled by the ventilator, there is then time for the bronchodilating and steroidal medications to work. The ventilator may be necessary for several days, although this varies depending on the patient's progress. There is no question that if a patient requires mechanical ventilation, his prognosis remains somewhat guarded over the next few days. Generally speaking, the outlook can still be quite good if there is sufficient time to initiate mechanical ventilation before the occurrence of any complications, such as irregular heartbeats or prolonged oxygen deprivation.

Avoiding a Recurrence of Status Asthmaticus. In most cases of status asthmaticus, there is usually a reason asthma symptoms became so out of control. By far the major cause of difficult-to-manage asthma is failure to identify and to manage asthma symptoms early enough. As a result, symptoms become so severe that the patient's normal back-up medications, or even medications routinely used in the emergency room, prove unrewarding. This sequence of events makes clear why it is so important to develop a close working relationship with a doctor who feels comfortable treating asthma, and to call the doctor early on if your normal backup medications do not provide relief. *THE IMPORTANCE OF EARLY TREATMENT OF ASTHMA SYMPTOMS CANNOT BE OVEREMPHASIZED*, for asthma symptoms that are neglected can progress to a potentially life-threatening point.

Asthma symptoms usually begin gradually and, if left untreated, increase in intensity during the course of several hours or several days. You are the exception if your initial asthma symptoms are sudden and severe. A careful review of your medical history is important to rule out the possibility that your sudden asthma flares could be caused by aspirin and aspirin-containing products (page 32), nonsteroidal anti-inflammatory medications (page 34), yellow food dye #5, or sulfites (page 47). The potential of an environmental or an occupational exposure must also be considered. If you have severe asthma attacks that begin suddenly without warning, you should have a medication program available that directs you to one or two steps that you can take immediately.

Essential steps to be taken by anyone who recently was

treated for status asthmaticus include: (a) understanding what happens during an asthma attack; (b) identifying and avoiding the particular factors that trigger your asthma symptoms; (c) writing down and following the exact timing and dose of the asthma medications prescribed by your doctor; (d) being certain that you understand how to use each of your medications properly, such as an inhaler; (e) being certain that you understand how to use back-up medications if your routine medication program fails to control your asthma; and (f) notifying your doctor immediately if the back-up medications are not helpful so that additional medications can be tried, in the hope of avoiding emergency room treatment.

Status asthmaticus is a potentially life-threatening condition, but it is often avoidable for most asthma patients.

SUMMARY: STATUS ASTHMATICUS

1. Status asthmaticus is a severe, potentially life-threatening asthma episode that initially fails to respond to routine medication treatment, including Adrenalin (when given by injection up to three times, spaced by twenty minutes), theophylline (when given intravenously), and/or bronchodilating solutions (with a nebulizer).

2. The normal response of the body when the airways are blocked during status asthmaticus is to increase the rate of breathing. This increases the oxygen and decreases the carbon dioxide level in the blood. However, when inflammation and obstruction of the airways become severe and the patient becomes fatigued from the work of breathing, the oxygen can decrease and the carbon dioxide can increase in the bloodstream. If this should occur, it may be necessary to support the patient's breathing by mechanical ventilation. For this reason physicians monitor the oxygen and carbon dioxide levels in the patient's arterial blood (an arterial blood-gas test) during a severe asthma attack.

3. In most cases of status asthmaticus there is usually a

reason asthma symptoms became so out of control. Typical factors include forgetting to take medications, neglecting to call the doctor early enough, and ignoring asthma symptoms in the hope that they will improve on their own. Asthma symptoms that rapidly become severe (within hours) can also be caused by products that contain aspirin or cross-react with aspirin, or by products that contain sodium metabisulfite. Although asthma symptoms usually become progressively worse over several days, there is a small group of patients whose asthma begins quite rapidly. This is more commonly the case with children. When an asthma management plan is formulated for someone with rapid onset of asthma symptoms, this factor must be taken into account.

4. Asthma can at times be so severe that wheezing is not heard, since there is not enough air movement in and out of the chest to produce a wheezing sound.

5. Treatment of status asthmaticus is similar to routine asthma treatment but is more intensive. Your pulse, heart rhythm, and respiratory rate are carefully monitored. Intravenous medications are used rather than oral medications. Inhalation treatments are given with a nebulizer using a bronchodilating solution every two hours, as long as the pulse rate is not excessively elevated. High doses of steroids are administered intravenously on a frequent basis (every four to six hours). Supplemental oxygen is used to increase the amount of oxygen that reaches your airways.

6. Be certain that you inform the doctor caring for your asthma of any medical problems you may have, such as heart, thyroid, or blood pressure problems.

7. Sedatives must be avoided during status asthmaticus, since they can suppress the rate of breathing and the urge to breathe.

8. Inhalation medications are best administered with a neb-

ulizer, as opposed to an IPPB machine, which delivers the medications under pressure to the airways. The pressure from IPPB machines may result in injury to the lung such as a pneumothorax (which occurs when air escapes from the airways or air sacs into the chest cavity).

9. During status asthmaticus, the blood theophylline level is frequently checked to be sure that it is within therapeutic range (10 to 20 micrograms per milliliter of blood serum). Adjustments in the dose of theophylline are made if you are taking a medication that affects the body's metabolism of theophylline, if you have heart or liver problems, or if you routinely take theophylline.

10. Steroids are essential during status asthmaticus. *IT WOULD BE A MISTAKE TO WITHHOLD STEROIDS DURING STATUS ASTHMATICUS FOR FEAR OF STEROID DEPENDENCY OR STEROID SIDE EFFECTS*, for these risks are associated with long-term, not the short-term, use of steroids.

11. If the management approach outlined above proves unrewarding, and/or the patient becomes fatigued from the effort of breathing, a breathing tube is inserted in the patient's airway so that a machine can take over the work of breathing for the patient. When mechanical ventilation is required, the patient's prognosis remains somewhat guarded over the next few days, but the outlook for the recovery of most patients is still quite good.

12. The goal once asthma symptoms are under control is to avoid a recurrence of status asthmaticus and the need for hospitalization. Above all else, *EARLY TREATMENT OF ASTHMA SYMPTOMS IS A MUST*. Although status asthmaticus is a potentially life-threatening condition, it is usually avoidable for most asthma sufferers.

PART FIVE

◇◇◇◇◇

Special Problems

◇ 14 ◇

Difficult-to-Manage Asthma

In contrast to the 1950s, asthma-related deaths in the United States today are quite rare. Yet each year an estimated two thousand to four thousand asthma-related deaths occur in the United States. Since asthma is described as obstructive airway disease that is reversible, it is tragic when asthma becomes so out of control that the asthma patient dies. It is therefore important to understand the factors that can lead to asthma symptoms that are difficult to manage.

Key factors that place a patient at greater risk include: (a) severe asthma flares that begin suddenly; (b) delay in seeking care by ignoring or failing to recognize the severity of the attack and assuming that the asthma symptoms will resolve on their own; (c) noncompliance with the medication program suggested by the doctor, despite routine daily asthma symptoms; (d) failure to utilize recommended back-up medications when asthma symptoms flare; or (e) failure to notify the doctor early when the suggested regimen is not sufficient.

You Are Part of the Asthma Management Team.
Needless to say, ideal asthma care requires a working relationship between doctor and patient. As important as it is for the doctor to correctly assess the medication needs of the patient, it is equally important for the patient to realize that

he or she is an important part of the management team. If you tend to downplay your asthma and to take prescribed medications randomly rather than as directed, discuss this with your doctor. In addition, if you panic and become frightened when your asthma flares, your doctor must know this.

Construct a Written Medication Schedule Using Your Doctor's Suggestions. The sample medication programs reviewed in Chapter 5 emphasize the importance of understanding the proper dosage and timing of all of your medications. This allows you to avoid confusion and to get the fullest benefit from the prescribed medications. You should construct a medication outline similar to the sample programs, using the medications prescribed by your doctor. Once you have the program on paper, bring it to your doctor to be sure that it is accurate and complete. Above all, your program should include instructions about when to call your doctor and what to use for a back-up medication in the event that your routine medications prove unrewarding.

Aspirin-Containing Products as a Cause of Severe Asthma Flares. Sudden asthma flares that are quite difficult to manage can occur in patients sensitive to aspirin. Some studies report that as many as one out of every five asthma patients experiences a significant drop in the ability to breathe after taking aspirin, regardless of prior history with aspirin intake. It has been reported that patients who are sensitive to aspirin may also be sensitive to the nonsteroidal anti-inflammatory medications such as ibuprofen (Motrin), naproxen (Naprosyn), and piroxicam (Feldene). Aspirin-sensitive individuals may also be sensitive to indomethacin (Indocin), phenylbutazone (Butazolidin), and tartrazine (yellow food dye #5). (See Table 2–4 for a list of cross-reacting drugs.) Strict avoidance of these medications by patients who have nasal polyps is a must. It can be argued that all asthma patients, regardless of prior experience with aspirin, should avoid aspirin and aspirin-containing products as well as the medications listed above. You should review this question with your doctor.

If you are sensitive to aspirin, all aspirin and aspirin-containing products should be avoided (see Table 2–3). It is important to be a careful label reader, as aspirin is found in a number of products where it is not indicated in the name of the product. As an alternative to aspirin, acetaminophen (Tylenol) appears to be acceptable for most people (see Table 2–5). If stronger medication is required to manage arthritis or other medical problems associated with pain, review the proposed medication with the doctor managing your asthma before you start taking the new medication.

Checking Your Breathing at Home. If you have difficulty determining how well or poorly you are breathing, there is a device available for home use that can measure your lung function (breathing status). This device is called a peak-flow meter. If you have daily asthma symptoms or if your asthma attacks come on suddenly, objective confirmation with serial daily measurements of your peak-flow may prove useful to indicate when you need to seek medical attention. Peak-flow meters for home use are available from surgical supply houses without prescription. However, you should review the proper use of the peak-flow meter with your doctor.

Do You Follow Your Doctor's Instructions? It is essential that you be frank with yourself. If you have the tendency to make little of your asthma symptoms, counting on the fact that they will subside with time, you are taking far too great a risk. It is important to you and your doctor to establish a written medication and management schedule. Once the program is established, it is your responsibility to take an active role by following the program and notifying your doctor if it does not work. Management of a chronic illness such as asthma requires that the doctor and patient work together.

Your Psychological Status Is Equally Important. Asthma care is not limited to medication programs, avoidance techniques, allergy shots and the like. The doctor must also understand the psychological status of his patient. Although asthma is not a psychosomatic illness, asthma can certainly be made worse by underlying psychological problems. In addition, many asthma patients have increased ''panic-fear'' levels associated with their asthma symptoms. Oftentimes, emotional support ranging from relaxation techniques to psychiatric counseling can be quite helpful in coping with asthma. You should be honest with your doctor so that he can best determine if the emotional aspect of your problem should be addressed. If counseling is suggested, try to be open-minded to the idea—your doctor is thinking of you as a person and not just as an asthmatic. See Chapter 12, ''Psychological Aspects.''

Potential Factors That Can Lead to Severe Asthma Problems. Other factors that, in the extreme case, may lead to death in some individuals include gross abuse of inhaled bronchodilators, sudden stopping or rapid tapering of steroids in steroid-dependent patients, and other complicating problems such as lung collapse. It is *imperative* that you follow the specific instructions of your doctor and keep him informed of your progress.

Inhalers should never be used excessively. If you need to use your inhaler more frequently than prescribed, that is a signal to contact your doctor. It is foolish to assume that repeated doses of the inhaler will bail you out of trouble. By far the greatest concern with inhaler overuse is that it causes delay in seeking medical care, although the potential also exists for causing irregular heartbeats. In addition, if routine use of your inhaler seems to make your condition worse, notify your doctor. This is a rare situation called a paradoxical response. Above all, do not neglect your asthma symptoms when a simple phone call to your doctor can more often than not resolve the situation.

All changes in steroid dosing should be determined by your doctor. It would be an error for you to take the lead in determining your steroid dose. Do not abruptly stop taking steroids out of frustration or out of concern for side effects. Remember that additional steroids are needed in times of stress. If you are worried about the potential of side effects from steroids, discuss the issue with your doctor. Remember that steroid side effects occur as a result of long-term (not short-term) use of steroids. Therefore, continuing steroids as directed by your doctor for a few additional days until you can arrange an office visit will not, in all probability, increase the risk of steroid side effects.

Increased Mucus Production Can Make Asthma More Difficult to Manage. Production of large amounts of mucus within the airways can be a major factor in making asthma more difficult to manage in some patients. The quantity of mucus coughed up can at times be truly astounding—as much as several cups per day. This mucus can clog the airways and make breathing more difficult, and can also serve as a source of infection.

In this setting, clearing of mucus and attention to the potential of an underlying infection are important. Antibiotics are often prescribed if it appears that mucus plugs within the airway have become infected. Bronchodilators are helpful for opening the airways to allow mucus to be more readily cleared. Steroids are usually essential when mucus production is excessive, as they help to reduce mucus secretion and reduce inflammation within the airways.

Practical approaches such as increasing clear fluid intake and inhaling steam can also be of benefit. A valuable physical therapy approach is percussion and postural drainage, in which various areas of the back and chest are firmly tapped and vibrated while you sit or recline in specific positions. This allows mucus to be loosened and then to be cleared or coughed out of the airways. Percussion and postural drainage are usually performed shortly after using your bronchodilating inhaled medication.

Percussion and postural drainage should only be done by someone who has been trained to perform this technique properly. Done incorrectly, it can fracture a rib or create other complications. If excessive mucus production is a chronic problem, family members and friends can be taught to perform percussion and postural drainage for you at home.

Percussion and postural drainage should not be performed during an acute asthma flare. If your medication program is not sufficient to control your asthma symptoms, notify your doctor. Discuss whether percussion and postural drainage would be helpful for you in nonemergency situations.

Complications of Asthma. If your symptoms are different from usual, you should notify your doctor. There is the possibility that another problem could be complicating your asthma.

Look for a marked worsening of shortness of breath, chest pain located on one side only, or a cough that produces discolored mucus in association with a fever. Complications of asthma can include rib fractures as a result of extensive coughing, escape of air from the airways into the chest (pneumothorax) which can occur without reason, as well as collapse of a portion of the lung, often due to mucus plugging the airways (atelectasis). By far the most frequent complication is infection, ranging from an infection of mucus plugs that are trapped behind blocked airways to pneumonia. A complication may be the reason why your body sometimes doesn't respond to treatment during an acute asthma attack. A chest X-ray is of value if your doctor needs to determine whether there are any complications related to your asthma symptoms.

Avoid Sleeping Medications When Asthma Flares. When your asthma is acting up, you should not use sleeping medications, as they can suppress your breathing and lead to a worsening of your problem. When you are short of breath, it is essential that you breathe to the fullest of your ability. When you are sleepy, you cannot work as hard to breathe and to help clear your airways. Although it might seem that a good night of sleep would be desirable, it could be a critical mistake to take sleeping medications when asthma symptoms flare.

Final Points to Consider in Coping with Difficult Asthma. It would be helpful for you to review the sample programs #8 to #11 (page 169), which pertain to difficult-to-manage asthma. In addition, a series of questions that you should answer is presented in Table 14–1. By being well informed and seeking medical attention early, you can considerably reduce the risk of complications.

SUMMARY: DIFFICULT-TO-MANAGE ASTHMA

1. Deaths caused by asthma are rare but do occur. Oftentimes, these deaths could have been prevented. It is important to understand the factors that can place a person with asthma at greater risk.

Points to Consider in Managing Difficult Asthma

1. Are there any special factors in your asthma case history that have not been addressed such as sinusitis, gastroesophageal reflux, or cardiac asthma?

2. Are you using your medications properly such as proper inhaler technique, proper sequence and spacing of medications?

3. Do you need a nebulizer for use at home to open your airways for routine or emergency treatment?

4. Has the dose and timing of your theophylline been checked to be sure it is within the therapeutic range and does not drop between doses?

5. Are you a candidate for a preventative medication such as cromolyn sodium or an inhaled steroid?

6. If you require oral steroids on a routine basis, are they used in as ideal a manner as possible? (see page 110)

7. If you require oral steroids on a routine basis, are you a candidate for one of the lesser known medications such as atropine or TaO? (Note that these medications should be used only under the supervision of an asthma specialist.)

8. Have you discussed with your doctor whether you should obtain a second opinion or visit an asthma treatment center?

Table 14–1

2. You are part of the asthma management team. As such, you must notify your doctor early when your recommended medications are not working. Do not ignore asthma symptoms that fail to respond to recommended medications.

3. Prescribed medications must be taken as directed and on time. Taking routine medications only when you remember can increase your risk of an asthma flare. In addition, this practice is a forerunner to neglecting your asthma

symptoms so that they are allowed to progress and become more serious.

4. Be frank with your doctor. If you get so nervous when you have asthma symptoms that you fail to follow instructions, your doctor should know this. If you ignore symptoms as a way of denying that you have asthma, tell your doctor so that consideration can be given to psychological support.

5. Do not break any of the rules recommended by your doctor. Suggestions include: (a) Do not take any sleeping medications when your breathing status is not perfect. (b) Never use your inhaler more than the prescribed amount without notifying your doctor. (c) Never taper off or stop steroid dosages on your own—only your doctor can change your steroid treatment. (d) Notify your doctor if your symptoms are in any way different from usual. (e) Carefully check product labels if you are supposed to avoid aspirin-containing products, nonsteroidal anti-inflammatories, tartrazine (yellow food dye #5), or sulfites.

6. Extensive mucus production within the airways can make breathing more difficult and also serve as a source of infection. Therapy can include medications (such as bronchodilators, antibiotics, and steroids), physical therapy (percussion and postural drainage), as well as practical suggestions (increased fluid intake and use of inhaled steam).

7. Write down all of your doctor's suggestions. Set up a medication program similar to the sample programs in Chapter 5, using the medications prescribed by your doctor. Review this chart with your doctor so that any misunderstandings can be clarified.

8. Table 14–1 highlights some points to consider in managing difficult asthma.

◇ 15 ◇

Asthma Flares at Night

Asthma symptoms tend to occur at night and in the early morning hours. This can be quite annoying for the asthma patient as it often disturbs a night of sleep. In addition, flares of asthma that are severe also are more likely to occur at night or early in the morning. People who have nighttime asthma symptoms may have little or no asthma symptoms during the day. The reason many people have increased asthma symptoms at night is not yet fully understood. Although treatment of nighttime asthma can be difficult, a practical approach can help make the asthma sufferer more comfortable at night.

Long-Acting Theophylline Is the Preferred Agent for Routine Nighttime Symptoms. The first step is to identify whether this is the most likely time of day for you to have symptoms. If you have noticed a worsening of asthma symptoms at night, mention this to your doctor. The medications that have proved to be of most benefit in this situation are long-acting theophylline preparations such as Theo-dur or Slo-bid (see Table 3–5). The timing of your dose of medication can also be important. For most people with nighttime asthma flares, a dosing schedule of 10:00 A.M. and 10:00 P.M. makes sense. With this schedule, the theophylline is at its peak in the early morning hours, when asthma symptoms are most likely to occur. As back-up to the theophylline product, a longer-acting inhaled bronchodilator such as albuterol should be available. Two puffs of the inhaler (spaced by five minutes) can be of great benefit.

Cromolyn as a Pretreatment for Environmental Allergens. When environmental factors such as exposure to pets seem to be a major precipitant of nighttime asthma symptoms, cromolyn sodium (Intal) can be used as a pretreatment regimen by itself or in combination with a long-acting theophylline product. For example, if your asthma is triggered by your pet, using cromolyn twenty minutes prior to entering your house and again at bedtime may prove sufficient to block asthma symptoms. Prior to using cromolyn, a bronchodilating inhaler can be used to open the airways to allow the cromolyn better access to the airways. Even if cromolyn is not used routinely during the day, the use of cromolyn in this manner may be quite helpful in managing nighttime asthma symptoms.

Bronchodilating Inhalers Are Usually Sufficient for Occasional Nighttime Asthma. For those individuals who have this problem only occasionally, it is usually sufficient to have on hand a bronchodilating inhaler to use as needed. If you wake up during the night with asthma symptoms, you can use two puffs of the inhaler, spaced by five minutes. For individuals with mild asthma symptoms, this usually allows them to get back to sleep.

Steroids Are the Last Alternative for Nighttime Asthma. Steroids are sometimes used to treat nighttime asthma in combination with an inhaled bronchodilator and a long-acting theophylline product. As is the general rule, steroids should be used as a last alternative and should be administered as ideally as possible (see page 110). Use of steroids at night to block asthma should be avoided if at all possible. For many patients, a combination of medications can avoid the need for steroids.

Environmental Precautions Are Worthwhile. Attention to environmental allergens, especially in the bedroom, can make a difference for many people. Allergens such as dust, mold, animal danders, and feather pillows are typical year-round culprits. If you sleep with your bedroom windows open during the pollen seasons, pollens can enter the bedroom and trigger asthma symptoms. Even if you are not allergic, environmental allergens can serve as irritants to the airways and bring on asthma symptoms. Suggestions for keeping your environment, and your bedroom in particular, as free as possible of potential irritants and allergens can be found in Chapter 6, which discusses precautions for limiting dust and mold exposure. Simple maneuvers such as using a bedspread during the day to prevent dust from collecting on pillows and bedding and then removing the bedspread at night so that you are not exposed to the dust can be quite helpful.

One allergen that might play a role in nighttime asthma flares is the house-dust mite. House-dust mites are microscopic organisms which can be a component of house dust. The mite is invisible to the naked eye, measuring only 0.2 millimeters in length, and feeds on food particles, scales from human skin, and other debris. As we all shed these scales during the course of the day, mites have abundant feeding material in the home. Mattresses, sofas, and upholstered chairs are particular sites for mite growth and proliferation. Studies have shown that when an asthma patient is exposed to house-dust mites, the patient's breathing status can drop. Since house-dust mites live in bedding and mattresses, the house-dust mite may well be one of the culprits in nighttime asthma flares. As mites prefer cooler temperatures and a damp environment, you should wash your bedding in hot water rather than cold in order to eliminate house-dust mites as much as possible.

Nasal Congestion and Postnasal Drip May Contribute to Nighttime Asthma. In addition to asthma medications and environmental precautions, another approach that may help to improve nighttime asthma flares is to treat nasal symptoms such as postnasal drip. Mucus that drips to the back of the throat may stimulate irritant receptors located there which are capable of triggering the airways to constrict, thereby leading to asthma symptoms. Use of an antihistamine and/or a decongestant at night may prove helpful, as long as your asthma symptoms are not made worse by the dryness of the airways these products infrequently cause. Also, inhaled steroids such as beclomethasone (Vancenase or Beconase) or flunisolide (Nasalide) can be used for a one-week trial period to see if nighttime symptoms improve.

Other Potential Causes of Nighttime Asthma. Other factors currently being explored as possible explanations for nighttime asthma include : (a) cooling of the airways which occurs during sleep; (b) passage of digestive products from the stomach into the airways, which can occur in the reclined position in a small group of individuals (see gastroesophageal reflux, page 282); and (c) variation in the tension of the muscles surrounding the airways, with increased airway constriction apparently occurring at night.

Although the normal pattern for steroid secretion results in a drop in steroid secretion at night, this does not, on its own, appear to explain nighttime asthma flares. When supplemental steroids are given at night during scientific studies, nighttime asthma is not necessarily prevented. A normal nighttime drop in the circulating Adrenalin may also contribute to the complexity of nighttime asthma symptoms.

SUMMARY: ASTHMA SYMPTOMS AT NIGHT

1. A clear-cut explanation of why asthma symptoms tend to flare at night and in the early morning hours is not yet available.

2. It is important to identify whether this is the most likely time for you to have asthma symptoms so that appropriate therapy can be prescribed.

3. Long-acting theophylline is the preferable medication if nighttime asthma flares occur routinely. For intermittent symptoms, inhaled bronchodilators can be taken prior to

bedtime or when symptoms occur. Cromolyn sodium can also be tried as a pretreatment for nighttime asthma. Steroids should be the last alternative. Your response to the prescribed medication should be reviewed with your doctor.

4. Precautions against environmental allergens should not be neglected. The bedroom must be as free as possible of allergens and irritants.

5. Consideration should also be given to the possibility that nighttime asthma flares could be caused by postnasal drip from allergic or sinus problems, or reflux of material from the stomach into the airways.

Gastroesophageal Reflux

The term gastroesophageal reflux means that some of the liquid, acidic contents of the stomach pass, in the wrong direction, up the feeding tube (the esophagus). This material can irritate the esophagus and cause it to become inflamed. If any of the material passes further up the esophagus and then accidentally passes into the airways, it can serve as an irritant and trigger asthma flares. This possibility should be considered if you have difficult-to-manage asthma. If you tend to belch up acidic stomach contents, have heartburn, or have a history of a hiatus hernia (although you can have reflux without a hiatal hernia), discuss this with your doctor, as this information should be added to your records.

Reflux is most likely to occur at night, since we sleep in a reclined position which allows passage of the liquid material from the stomach up into the esophagus. A muscle called the lower esophageal sphincter normally prevents contents of the stomach from passing up into the esophagus. Those individuals with the tendency toward reflux have an incompetent sphincter. Often there are no clues that this condition exists other than troublesome asthma symptoms, especially at night.

An upper gastrointestinal X-ray (UGI series) can identify if you have a hiatal hernia and, at times, show reflux. The radiologist who performs the UGI series might be able to detect the passage of stomach contents into the esophagus, confirming the diagnosis of reflux. However, the chances are small that reflux into the airways themselves could be demonstrated by X-ray. The presence of reflux into the esophagus alone is reason for treatment of this condition in someone who has difficult asthma, as therapy directed to this problem may improve asthma symptoms.

Medical management of reflux consists of: (a) elevating the head of the bed at night; (b) eating smaller and, if necessary, more frequent meals, so that the stomach does not become overly full; (c) eliminating any eating within three hours of bedtime; and (d) using antacids two hours after eating and at bedtime, to buffer the acidity of stomach contents so that they are less irritating. Other alternatives can be considered such as the use of cimetidine (Tagamet) or ranitidine (Zantac), which reduce the acid secretion of the stomach. Weight reduction and cessation of alcohol and cigarettes, when applicable, are also important.

Interestingly, theophylline has a tendency to loosen the lower esophageal sphincter. In individuals who are susceptible to reflux, the use of theophylline can increase the chance that reflux will occur. If you have a tendency toward reflux, your doctor may at times find it necessary to reduce your nighttime theophylline dose and support your asthma with other medications such as an inhaled bronchodilator by itself or along with an inhaled steroid such as beclomethasone (Vanceril) or triamcinolone (Azmacort). However, the benefit derived from theophylline in controlling asthma symptoms often outweighs the small chance that theophylline will be the predominant factor in triggering reflux. You should rely on your doctor's judgment in this regard.

If the medical management outlined above proves unrewarding, consideration can be given to a surgical approach to the problem. As surgery for gastroesophageal reflux is extensive and is not successful for everyone, it seems reasonable to undergo an extensive trial of medical management before considering an operation.

Since gastroesophageal reflux can make asthma symptoms more difficult to treat, you should discuss this possibility with your doctor if you have any of the symptoms discussed above.

SUMMARY: GASTROESOPHAGEAL REFLUX

1. When liquid contents from the stomach pass, in the wrong direction, up the esophagus, this is called gastroesophageal reflux. If this material gets into the airways, it can act as an irritant and trigger an asthma flare.

2. Gastroesophageal reflux can be an explanation for asthma that is difficult to manage.

3. If you have a hiatus hernia or symptoms such as belching, your doctor should be aware of this, although it is possible to have reflux without any symptoms. Asthma flares caused by reflux tend to occur during the night, as the reclined position favors reflux.

4. An upper gastrointestinal X-ray (UGI series) can help diagnose gastroesophageal reflux.

5. Medical management of the problem is preferable, as surgery for reflux is a major procedure and is not always successful. Suggestions for medical management are outlined in this chapter.

◇ 17 ◇

The Impact of the Upper Airway (Nose and Sinuses) on Asthma

It has become increasingly clear to physicians who treat asthma that problems in the upper airway (the nose and the sinuses) can have impact on the lower airway (the breathing tubes). If your nose is congested or if you have an underlying sinus infection, it is possible that your asthma symptoms will flare. As emphasized throughout this book, attention to details can make a great difference in how you feel. It is important not to ignore nasal and sinus symptoms or to assume that they are simply a nuisance that need not be treated.

Irritant Receptors in Back of Throat Can Trigger Asthma Flares. The mechanism explaining how upper airway problems can cause asthma symptoms is still a matter of debate among doctors. However, it is clear that nerves that go from the nose and sinuses to the air tubes can trigger an asthma response. In addition, when the sinuses are congested, sinus secretions drain toward the back of the throat. The normal response is then to try to clear the secretions by clearing one's throat. The presence of the secretions in the back of the throat and the actual clearing of the throat can stimulate irritant receptors located in the back of the throat. Stimulation of these irritant receptors can trigger the air tubes to constrict, thereby causing asthma symptoms to flare.

285

Proper Management of Nasal and Sinus Symptoms Can Improve Asthma Symptoms. Regardless of the reasons, it is clear that medical treatment of upper airway symptoms can result in a surprising degree of improvement in your asthma symptoms. When someone has difficult-to-manage asthma that is unresponsive to medications, there is value in checking the sinuses by X-ray or sending the patient to an otolaryngologist (ear, nose, and throat specialist) for a careful check-up. In comparison to the difficulty involved with asthma symptoms, the added problem of a stuffy nose often is regarded by patients as unimportant. Yet improvement in your nasal or sinus symptoms can sometimes bring about the improvement in your asthma that you have been hoping for. In view of this, it is worthwhile to review the function of the nose and the problems that can cause nasal congestion.

The Functions of the Nose. The nose functions as a filter to keep foreign particles from entering our airways. In addition, the nose warms and humidifies the air before it enters the lower airways. These functions require the presence of some degree of mucus and congestion in the nose. The balance between keeping the nose open as opposed to congested is under the control of nerves supplied to the area.

A. ALLERGIC RHINITIS

Allergic rhinitis is the medical term used to describe the nasal congestion, runny nose, and sneezing that result from exposure to something to which you are allergic. Allergies can also be responsible for itchy, watery eyes (allergic conjunctivitis) and asthma symptoms (allergic asthma). Allergic rhinitis can occur on a year-round basis (perennial allergic rhinitis) or follow a seasonal pattern (seasonal allergic rhinitis, or hay fever).

Seasonal Allergic Rhinitis. Seasonal allergic rhinitis is an allergic reaction to seasonal pollens affecting the nose. The classic example is ragweed allergy. Ragweed pollinates in many parts of the United States during the later part of the summer and early fall and is responsible for causing nasal, eye, and chest symptoms in millions of sensitive individuals. The term "hay fever" is a misnomer for nasal allergies, as hay is not the culprit and sufferers do not typically have fever. Despite the misnomer, the term "hay fever" commonly is used to describe the medical term "seasonal allergic rhinitis."

Perennial Allergic Rhinitis. Perennial allergic rhinitis is usually caused by allergens such as house dust, house-dust mites, molds, animal danders (typically from dogs and cats), and feathers. For the person with perennial allergic rhinitis, nasal symptoms persist throughout the year rather than varying from season to season.

Frequency of Allergic Nasal Symptoms. It is estimated that approximately fifteen million Americans suffer from allergic nasal symptoms. Symptoms can occur at any age but children and young adults are more likely to be affected. The incidence of allergic nasal symptoms tends to decrease in older age groups. Although the tendency to develop allergies is hereditary, the development of allergies does require prior exposure to a potential allergen over time. Typically a patient has two or three years of exposure to a new area of the country or to a new pet at home before nasal symptoms become severe enough to prompt an allergy evaluation.

How Allergies Cause Nasal Symptoms. As previously discussed (page 16), allergy symptoms occur when an individual with an inherited tendency to develop allergies is exposed to a potential allergen such as ragweed or house dust. With time, the allergic individual develops antibodies called IgE that are specifically directed to the allergen(s) to which the person is allergic. These IgE antibodies become attached to mast cells located in the nose, skin, breathing tubes, and conjunctiva of the eyes. When the IgE antibodies come in contact with the specific allergens to which they are directed, the mast cells release chemicals such as histamine which cause allergy symptoms. When this process occurs in the nose, the symptoms are called allergic rhinitis. When this process occurs in the eyes, it is called allergic conjunctivitis, and in the airways, allergic asthma.

Airborne Pollens Cause Seasonal Allergic Rhinitis.

As noted earlier, the nasal symptoms typical of seasonal allergic rhinitis are caused by lightweight pollens from plants that depend on the wind for pollination. Pollens from plants that depend on insects for pollination, such as goldenrod and dandelions, are too heavy to become airborne and therefore cause nasal symptoms only when you directly smell the plants. This distinction is important, as many people think that goldenrod, the gold-colored weed they see along the roadside in late summer and fall, is the trigger for their hay fever. However, this is not the case. Rather, the slender, candelabra-shaped ragweed plant, which is often found in the same area, is the major cause of allergic nasal, chest, and eye symptoms.

Know the Seasonal Pattern of Your Area.

If you notice that your nasal symptoms are worse at certain times of the year, you should compare this with the seasonal pollen pattern for your area. For example, in the eastern and midwestern parts of the United States, ragweed pollinates from mid-August until the first frost (usually around late October). Tree pollen is prevalent in the early part of the spring (March to May), while grass pollen appears during the latter part of the spring and into summer (May to early July). Mold spores can mimic this seasonal pattern, since they increase in numbers during warm, damp weather. Daily pollen counts often include mold counts as well. Allergy skin testing can identify your exact allergic sensitivity. See Appendix A for a pollen calendar of the United States.

Weather Conditions and Time of Day Can Affect Severity of Symptoms.

Ragweed is an example of a plant that releases its pollen in the early morning hours. The pollen is then carried by the wind. It thus makes sense to keep the bedroom windows closed when going to bed at night and, if necessary, to use air conditioning instead. Open windows on a breezy fall morning provide an ideal setting for allergy symptoms to flare. Rain tends to clear the ragweed pollen from the air but enhances mold growth, which can trigger allergy symptoms in mold-allergic individuals.

Year-Round Symptoms. Year-round allergy symptoms can be triggered by exposure to house dust, molds, feather pillows, down comforters, and animal dander. It is not unusual to have both seasonal and year-round allergy symptoms. Exposure to dust is increased when there are lots of objects and clutter in a room. Bookshelves filled with books are a typical place for dust to collect. Molds flourish wherever there is a warm, moist environment. Ideal locations for mold growth include humidifiers, air conditioning units, and soil at the base of plants. A review of environmental precautions for dust and molds is presented on page 189. Although dust precautions may seem time consuming, studies have confirmed that reduction of your environmental exposure to dust, especially in the bedroom, can reduce asthma symptoms.

Other Potential Factors That Can Cause Year-Round Nasal Symptoms. Exposure to allergens at work can trigger year-round nasal congestion. Often a helpful clue that this is the case is that your nasal symptoms are better over the weekend. Irritants such as cigarette smoke, air pollution, and newsprint can cause similar nasal symptoms by directly irritating the nose, but this is not an allergic response. Foods have been suggested as a potential cause of nasal congestion, although this issue is heavily debated among physicians. Some patients do notice that some of the mold-containing foods can trigger nasal and, at times, chest symptoms (see Table 2–7, page 46.) If you notice this to be the case, review this with your doctor and consider avoiding the foods in question.

Typical Symptoms of Allergic Rhinitis. Nasal congestion, runny nose, itchiness of the nose, and frequent sneezing episodes are the hallmarks of allergic rhinitis. The mucus from the nose is thin and clear, often flowing continuously. If the mucus is discolored (such as yellow or green), this suggests that you may have an infection. With allergic rhinitis, the mucus membranes of the nose are usually congested; this can put pressure on the opening of the sinuses, causing sinus pressure and headache. Nasal congestion from allergic rhinitis can also put pressure on the opening of the eustachian tube which leads to the ears, thereby causing pressure in the ears. In addition to nasal symptoms, the eyes may be quite itchy and runny and asthma symptoms may flare. Postnasal drip from allergic rhinitis can also cause subtle chest symptoms (such as a dry, hacking cough) which can be mistaken for asthma symptoms.

Allergic Rhinitis and Asthma Involve the Same Mechanism but a Different Target Organ. Remember that the same mechanism that causes the nose to be congested with allergic rhinitis can also cause asthma symptoms. Namely, the mechanism involving the mast cells and specific IgE antibodies can trigger nasal symptoms in certain individuals and chest symptoms in those individuals with the tendency toward asthma. For some individuals, both the nose and the airways are affected, while for others, only one organ is affected.

"Priming Effect" of Added Allergic and Irritant Exposure. When, for a prolonged period, you are exposed to and experience symptoms from an allergen to which you are sensitive, your nose becomes "primed," ready to respond to irritants or to other allergens to which you are normally less sensitive. For example, when you are having nasal symptoms during the ragweed season and are then exposed to dust, the dust can trigger a worsening of your allergy symptoms even if you are normally not very sensitive to dust.

The Allergic Appearance. People who have allergies often breathe through their mouths and frequently itch or rub their noses. Allergic children often rub their noses in an upward and outward manner, similar to a salute, which has been called the "allergic salute." A crease may be present along the lower third of the nose as a result of frequent rubbing of the nose to relieve the itch. Dark circles may be present under the eyes, called "allergic shiners," and the eyes may appear quite red. When the doctor looks inside your nose, the mucus membranes are swollen and "boggy" and appear pale. If there is an infection in your nose the appearance is quite different, as the mucus membranes are then reddened.

How Doctors Diagnose Allergies. Allergies are diagnosed by a medical history suggesting a seasonal pattern or a particular exposure that makes symptoms worse. A review of your overall medical history and present medications allows your doctor to rule out other possibilities that may account for your symptoms. A careful physical examination is also important, looking for the characteristic appearance of the inside of the nose and checking for subtle asthma symptoms. Each of the other possible causes of chronic nasal congestion are considered during the course of the exam. Allergy skin tests are then performed.

Allergy Skin Tests. Allergy skin testing is performed to determine if someone is allergic. The doctor who performs the skin tests must carefully correlate the test results to the patient's medical history, as it is possible on occasion to have falsely positive or negative test results. Allergy skin testing identifies whether the specific allergy antibody for the allergen being tested is present on mast cells found in the patient's skin (see page 16).

There are two approaches to performing allergy skin tests—the scratch or prick test, and the intradermal test. The prick technique involves placing a drop of an extract of the allergen (such as dust, dog dander, or ragweed pollen) on the skin, typically on the back or forearm. Allergens are placed on the skin in rows so that multiple tests can be performed at the same time. A lancet is then used to gently scratch or puncture the skin to introduce the allergen into the skin. With the intradermal skin test, the allergen is injected in dilute form just under the skin to create a small bubble.

Within fifteen minutes of testing by either technique, a raised area called a wheal (like a hive or mosquito bite) surrounded by a reddish area called a flare will appear at the test site if the person is sensitive to that particular allergen. The tests are graded on a scale of 0 to 4 based on the size of the wheal and flare, with a 4+ reaction being the largest. If there is no change in the skin, the person is not sensitive to the tested allergen.

The prick test causes little discomfort and is quite safe (rarely causing an allergic reaction), as the allergen is simply placed on the skin. The intradermal test is like a tuberculin skin test and is slightly more uncomfortable, especially for small children. It has the advantage of being more sensitive than the prick test, but has a greater, although still small, risk of an allergic reaction. Allergic reactions to skin testing can range from redness of the face and itchiness of the skin to severe changes in blood pressure, with difficulty breathing, difficulty swallowing, and passing out. Fortunately these severe reactions are rare, but it is for this reason that allergists usually perform both tests together—starting with the prick test as a general screen followed by the intradermal test for those allergens that were negative by prick technique.

Allergy skin tests are compared to two controls—histamine (the end product of the allergic reaction) and saline. The histamine control checks to be certain that the skin's ability to react positively to an allergen has not been blocked by the patient's use of other medications. Antihistamines, for example, should not be used for one or two days before skin testing as they may block the test results. Asthma medications (including theophylline, the Adrenalin-like bronchodilators, and even steroids) do not block the allergy skin test results and therefore do not have to be withheld in preparation for skin testing. The saline control is used to identify patients who have sensitive skin which might give the false impression of positive skin test results.

Radioallergosorbent Test (RAST). The RAST is a blood test that measures the amount of specific IgE antibody in the patient's blood serum for the allergen that is tested. The RAST can be used in place of allergy skin testing as it provides information comparable to that provided by the intradermal skin test. The key advantage of RAST is that it involves drawing only a single blood sample from the patient; there is none of the discomfort associated with skin tests and no risk of reaction. It has practical application for young children (under three years old) as well as for patients who have skin problems, such as severe eczema, that would make skin testing impossible to interpret. However, the major disadvantages of RAST are that it is not as sensitive as skin testing and does not mirror as directly as skin testing what is happening in the body's tissues. Skin testing is also less expensive than RAST and offers results that can be interpreted immediately.

RAST results are on a scale of 0 to 6, with a score of 6 being clearly positive and 0 being clearly negative. Careful interpretation of test results is important for results that are not as clear-cut. Correlation of the test results with the patient's medical history is essential.

As of this writing, the American Academy of Allergy and Clinical Immunology recommends allergy skin testing instead of RAST testing in assessing one's allergy condition. Although some physicians are proponents of RAST rather than allergy skin tests, all of your allergy tests need to be interpreted by a physician trained in allergy.

Treatment of Allergic Nasal Symptoms. Management of allergic nasal symptoms includes avoidance suggestions for the particular allergen in question, judicious use of medication and, when appropriate, allergy immunotherapy (shots). Table 17-1 outlines the choices of medications available to date for treating allergic rhinitis, which include: (a) antihistamines which tend to dry nasal secretions, (b) decongestants which reduce the stuffiness of the nose, (c) topical nasal steroids which reduce inflammation within the nose and improve nasal symptoms, (d) nasal cromolyn sodium which may block the release of mediators such as histamine from the mast cell, and (e) oral steroids which are the last alternative and acceptable only for short-term use for allergic nasal symptoms.

Avoidance Techniques. The seasonal pollens are difficult to avoid since they are carried about by the wind. However, your exposure to the pollens can be reduced if you are aware of the seasonal pollination pattern in your area and the local daily pollen count, and if you use common sense in following suggestions for avoiding exposure to pollen as much as possible. Dust and mold avoidance around the house can also be

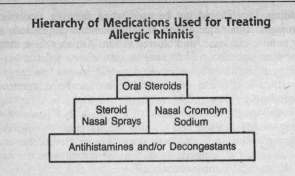

Hierarchy of Medications Used for Treating Allergic Rhinitis

Oral Steroids

Steroid Nasal Sprays | Nasal Cromolyn Sodium

Antihistamines and/or Decongestants

Antihistamines and/or decongestants are the most commonly used medications for managing allergic nasal symptoms. Steroid nasal sprays can be used short-term as a preventative if antihistamines prove unrewarding or cause sedating side effects which the patient cannot tolerate. Nasal cromolyn sodium is also a preventative medication and is typically free of side effects; however, it must be used frequently during the day. Oral steroids are rarely necessary for allergic rhinitis and should be reserved for short-term use only when absolutely necessary.

Table 17-1

quite challenging. Complete avoidance of dust and mold is not possible, yet there is value for sensitive patients in reducing exposure to dust and mold in the home. An approach to environmental precautions for the seasonal pollens, dust, and molds is presented in Chapter 6.

Medication Choices for Allergic Rhinitis

Antihistamines. The first step in managing allergy nasal symptoms is to try an antihistamine. A typical first choice is chlorpheniramine (Chlor-Trimeton) which is available over the counter. Antihistamines available by prescription are the next alternative. Since there are many good products, you should ask your doctor to let you try several so that you can find one that relieves your nasal symptoms but is not too sedating. Antihistamines are best taken only at bedtime, if possible, because they have the tendency to be sedating. In addition, they should not be used when drinking alcoholic beverages. Other side effects of antihistamines can include a dry mouth, dizziness, and blurred vision. At times these side effects are overcome when antihistamines are used continuously, but you should notify your doctor if you have any problems. Antihistamines should be used cautiously by patients who have a tendency toward urinary retention, as they can make this problem worse.

Decongestants. When nasal congestion is a problem, the addition of a decongestant such as pseudoephedrine (Sudafed) or Phenylpropanolamine (Propagest) or a combination product containing both an antihistamine and a decongestant should be considered. Side effects of the decongestants include increased heart rate, elevation of the blood pressure, and sleeplessness. If you have a tendency toward high blood pressure, your blood pressure must be closely followed while you are using decongestants. As emphasized previously, the topical nasal decongestant sprays available over the counter should be avoided.

Steroid Nasal Sprays. By far, some of the most important new medications available to doctors for managing allergic nasal symptoms are the steroid nasal sprays (also called topical steroid sprays). Some patients experience relief of nasal symptoms within hours of using a steroid nasal spray, while other patients notice improvement only after several days of use. These products differ from the over-the-counter sprays that contain nasal decongestants in that they do not cause rebound nasal congestion. The steroid nasal sprays available to date include: flunisolide (Nasalide), beclomethasone (Beconase and Vancenase), and dexamethasone (Decadron Nasal Turbinaire), Beclomethasone and flunisolide offer the advantage of being short-acting and rapidly metabolized so that there is little overall absorption into the body. Dexamethasone spray, on the other hand, is absorbed somewhat more by the body so that adrenal gland suppression can occur if used in excess. As a general rule, these products should be used on a short-term rather than a long-term basis. They can be quite helpful for relieving symptoms for several weeks during an allergy season. However, it has not been clearly established whether the steroid nasal sprays have any serious long-term consequences when used over a period longer than several months.

Nasal Cromolyn Sodium (Nasalcrom). Nasal cromolyn sodium is thought to block the mast cell's release of chemical mediators such as histamine. It is a preventative agent, blocking nasal symptoms when it is used routinely, and cannot offer immediate relief. Its advantages are that it can be used long-term since it does not contain steroid and is relatively free of side effects. However, it is quite short-acting and needs to be used four to six times a day. A nighttime antihistamine may be necessary for some individuals if the cromolyn does not provide relief throughout the night.

Oral Steroids, the Last Alternative. Oral steroids should be used only as the absolute last alternative for allergic nasal symptoms. If oral steroids are used, they should be used sparingly for the shortest time possible (no longer than a few days). Once the oral steroids bring allergic nasal symptoms under control, the use of antihistamines, decongestants, or nasal sprays (by prescription) should be considered for routine management.

Injected Steroids Are Best Avoided. Long-acting steroid preparations given by injection are best avoided because they carry an increased risk of steroid side effects. The availability of the steroid nasal sprays often makes steroid injections unnecessary for treatment of allergic rhinitis.

Allergy Immunotherapy Is Highly Successful for the Seasonal Pollens. Allergy shots contain small doses of the allergen to which you are allergic. They offer the potential that your allergy symptoms and your need for allergy medications can be reduced. Allergy shots make it possible for many individuals to go through an allergy season without the need for any medication. As opposed to medications that simply mask the symptoms, allergy shots actually reduce your sensitivity to the injected allergen.

Allergy shots for ragweed allergy have proved to be quite effective, with a success rate of up to 80 percent. The success rate for dust allergy is approximately 70 percent, while shots for mold allergy are somewhat controversial, with a more variable rate of success. The lower success rates for dust and mold allergies may be because there are many varieties of molds and many different components of dust. Ragweed, on the other hand, is but one allergen. Observations by many allergists suggest that allergy shots for dust along with avoidance of dust may prove more successful than either avoidance or medications alone. This point does, however, require further confirmation.

Candidates for Allergy Shots. Individuals are candidates for allergy shots if they have difficult-to-manage allergy symptoms that have not been controlled with medication alone or that require medication on a routine basis. These individuals usually have multiple, year-round allergies requiring daily medications. In addition, allergy shots can be considered for those who cannot tolerate the sedating effects of allergy nasal medications. Since the success of allergy shots depends on proper diagnosis of your allergies, your shot program should be developed and administered by a physician with training in the field of allergy.

The indications for the use of allergy shots for asthma patients, as well as a discussion of the mechanics and the risks of allergy shots, are presented in Chapter 7.

Other Causes of Chronic Nasal Congestion. When the nose is stuffy and runny on a routine basis, the usual explanation given is allergy. However, allergy is not the only cause of chronic nasal symptoms. A description is presented below of other potential causes which should be considered as possible reasons for routine nasal symptoms.

Abuse of Over-the-Counter Nasal Sprays Can Cause Rebound Nasal Congestion. Overuse and abuse of over-the-counter nasal sprays can aggravate the very symptoms they are designed to help. If over-the-counter nasal sprays such as Afrin, 4-Way, Dristan, and Neo-Synephrine are used for a prolonged period of time, the nose may eventually become stuffier, even though initially these medications open the nasal passageways by constricting the blood vessels within the mucus membranes of the nose. This phenomenon is called rebound nasal congestion and usually occurs after several or more days of use of the nasal spray. It is thus advisable to avoid products of this type (the list above is incomplete) as there is the tendency to allow their use to become a habit, despite warnings on the packages.

Other Medications Associated with Nasal Side Effects. On occasion, an oral medication you may be taking can be the culprit triggering increased nasal symptoms. Propranolol and reserpine are examples of medications that can cause nasal stuffiness. It is important that you carefully review with your asthma doctor all medications you are using.

Hormonal Influence on the Nose. Hormonal changes can have an impact on nasal congestion. The most common example is rhinitis of pregnancy, which is increased nasal congestion that typically begins late in the first trimester or in the second trimester and may continue until delivery. This condition is clearly not caused by allergy but can be made worse if you are allergic and are exposed to allergens. Another example of hormonal influence on nasal congestion is the increased nasal congestion that can be observed when the thyroid is underactive. Therefore, your doctor may want to check your thyroid status with blood tests if your nose remains congested on a routine basis.

Deviation of the Septum. Deviation of the nasal septum is an anatomical cause of nasal congestion. The two sides of the nose are separated by the nasal septum. When the septum is not lined up straight on the midline, this results in one of the nasal passageways being narrower than it should be. This deviation is quite common. It need not be corrected surgically unless it plays a role in increased nasal congestion that is quite uncomfortable and cannot otherwise be explained.

B. NASAL POLYPS

Nasal polyps are fluid-filled sacs that arise from the mucus membranes of the nose in some individuals. They frequently occur in individuals who have had chronic nasal or sinus problems, but also occur without clear-cut explanation. They are usually found in a small percentage of children with cystic fibrosis. Nasal polyps are not malignant. The biggest problem associated with polyps is that they block the nasal passageway, making breathing uncomfortable and sometimes causing lack of smell or taste.

Medical Treatment of Nasal Polyps. The treatment of nasal polyps can be difficult and can require the efforts of both your allergist and your otolaryngologist. A first step is often a trial of a topical nasal spray that contains steroid, such as beclomethasone (Beconase or Vancenase), flunisolide (Nasalide), or dexamethasone (Decadron Nasal Turbinaire). Antihistamines and decongestants can be tried but are often unsuccessful. Aspirin and aspirin-containing products as well as the cross-reacting medications (such as the nonsteroidal anti-inflammatories and yellow food dye #5) are best avoided. It is controversial whether there is any value in eliminating salicylates (found naturally in some foods) and yellow food dye #5 from your diet. Assessment of your allergies and treatment with environmental precautions to known allergens and allergy shots (when appropriate) can be worthwhile. Consideration can be given to the use of short courses of oral steroids to shrink the polyps, knowing that as the steroid dose is tapered down, the polyps may recur.

Surgical Treatment of Nasal Polyps. If this trial of medication is unsuccessful, and if the polyps continue to produce nasal obstruction that is troublesome, they can be removed surgically. However, there is a high rate of recurrence of nasal polyps after surgery, typically within six months, although they can recur at any time. Steroid nasal sprays can be used during the postoperative period and can be continued for several months if they are necessary to prevent the polyps from recurring. Although there is little steroid absorption into the body with beclomethasone and flunisolide, dexamethasone does carry a somewhat greater likelihood of causing suppression of the HPA axis (see page 107). Inhaled steroids should be used only under your doctor's supervision and should be used as infrequently as possible.

Oral Steroids Are the Last Alternative. For long-term use, oral steroids should be reserved as the last alternative, and then taken on a single morning or an alternate day dosage schedule. Efforts should be continued to use medications other than oral steroids to control nasal polyps. You must understand the risk of side effects associated with the long-term use of steroids (see page 109).

Avoid Aspirin-Containing Products and the Cross-Reacting Medications. If you have nasal polyps along with asthma, there is an increased chance that you could experience a severe, possibly life-threatening reaction to products that contain aspirin. All asthma patients who have nasal polyps should be aware of the association of nasal polyps, asthma, and aspirin sensitivity. This grouping is called triad asthma. Often asthma patients who have triad asthma also have sinusitis. If you have triad asthma, you should avoid all aspirin-containing and cross-reacting products (see Tables 2–3 and 2–4). All medications (especially pain relievers) should be reviewed with the doctor caring for your asthma before you take them. Severe asthma attacks can occur quite rapidly (within minutes) in patients who have triad asthma and inadvertently take aspirin or one of the medications that cross-react with aspirin.

Vasomotor Rhinitis. Vasomotor rhinitis is a catchall term for cases where there is no clear-cut allergic or other explanation for chronic nasal symptoms. This diagnosis implies that the nervous system's control of the nose is somehow altered, allowing the nose to remain congested. Typically, the patient notices that his nose becomes even more stuffy when he is exposed to changes in temperature or in barometric pressure, when he is under stress, or when he is exposed to noxious odors. Allergy skin testing is usually negative, and the various antihistamines and decongestants often fail to provide sustained relief. To date there is no single best option for this problem. Surgical approaches are generally unrewarding. A steroid nasal spray or cromolyn sodium (Nasalcrom) should be tried to see if the congestion improves.

C. SINUSITIS

Sinusitis is inflammation of the membranes lining the sinuses. Often the cause is an infection, although other possible causes should be considered, such as allergies, nasal polyps, a deviated nasal septum, swimming or diving, and abuse of nasal sprays. When the nose is congested, this can block the sinus openings into the nose, resulting in congestion and pressure within the sinuses. It is important for your nasal symptoms to be treated so as to lessen the risk of developing sinus complications. As mentioned previously, when the sinuses are congested or infected, asthma symptoms sometimes flare. Often by improving sinus symptoms, asthma symptoms improve so that less medication is needed for routine asthma management.

Location of the Sinuses. Figure 17–1 shows that the sinuses are air-filled cavities within the bones of the skull. Generally, the pain or headache associated with sinusitis occurs over the affected sinus area. However, it is possible for the pain from sinusitis to radiate to other areas of the head, thus making it more difficult to pinpoint the problem.

The Faulty Design of the Sinuses. The exact function of the sinuses is not clear-cut. When man assumed the upright posture, the sinuses no doubt helped to lessen the weight of the skull. One's sense of smell and the sound of one's voice are both influenced by the sinuses. Yet the design of the sinuses is less than ideal. For example, the maxillary sinus opening is located toward the top of the sinus, which makes it difficult for mucus secretions to drain from the sinuses. Another problem is that the maxillary sinus opening is po-

Location of the Sinuses

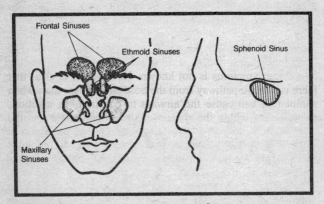

The maxillary sinuses are located over the cheekbones while the ethmoid sinuses are located on either side of the nose. The frontal sinuses are located above the eyes, across the forehead. The sphenoid sinus is located deeper within the skull.

Figure 17–1

sitioned in such a way that nasal congestion can block the sinus opening and interfere with sinus drainage even further.

Nasal Congestion Can Lead to Blockage of the Sinus Opening. When the nose is stuffy, the opening from the sinuses becomes blocked. Mucus within the sinus, which is normally cleared through the sinus opening, is then trapped in the sinus and becomes susceptible to infection. It is important to try to understand the reason for nasal congestion rather than to assume that sinus problems always stem from allergies or an infection such as a cold. A careful examination, checking for any anatomical obstruction such as deviation of the septum or nasal or sinus polyps, is an essential part of the doctor's evaluation of a patient with chronic sinus problems. Abuse of over-the-counter nasal decongestant sprays can be the cause of persistent nasal congestion. Flying, swimming, and diving should be avoided when you have sinus symptoms. With this understanding of the importance of decongesting the nose, it becomes apparent that the management of sinus problems involves not only treating any sinus infection but managing nasal congestion as well.

How Does Sinusitis Lead to Asthma Symptoms? The exact mechanism of how sinus problems trigger a worsening of asthma symptoms is not known. However, it is clear that there is a nerve pathway from the nose and sinuses that, when stimulated, can cause the airways to constrict. In addition, the infection within the sinuses can eventually extend to the back of the throat and the airways. Experience has shown that by reducing sinus symptoms either with medications or with surgery, improvement in asthma symptoms is likely to occur.

Symptoms Typical of Sinusitis. Sinusitis results in headache or pressure over the sinus area, along with nasal congestion and a change in mucus color to yellow or green (indicating an infection). Some individuals will experience headache alone. A sinus headache is often worse when bending over and when first getting up in the morning, and better when standing upright. Drainage occurs only if the sinus is open, so it is not unusual to have little drainage of infected sinus material. Fever may or may not occur even if there is an infection. Patients with long-standing sinusitis that has become chronic may have little or no symptoms typical of sinus problems. Therefore your doctor should check your sinuses as a possible source of chronic infection that could be a contributing factor to your asthma symptoms.

X-Ray Is an Important Diagnostic Tool. The diagnosis of sinusitis can be confirmed by obtaining an X-ray. This indicates whether there is any thickening of the walls of the sinuses. In addition, if there is an active infection, there may be fluid within the sinuses that can be detected by X-ray. Occasionally, an asthma patient without any history of sinus problems is given a sinus X-ray only to find that the patient does in fact have sinusitis. Therefore, it is not unusual for a doctor to obtain a sinus X-ray of a difficult-to-manage asthma patient who has no sinus symptoms.

Treatment of Sinusitis. The approach to sinusitis management is to decongest the nose to promote sinus drainage and to treat the infection.

Antibiotics for Sinusitis. If you are not allergic to penicillin, the preferable antibiotics for treating sinusitis are Ampicillin or Amoxicillin. Tetracycline, or trimethoprim-sulfamethoxazole (Septra or Bactrim) are the medications of choice if you are allergic to penicillin. The use of cephalosporins such as Keflex or Ceclor can be considered for treatment of sinusitis, although there is a 10 to 20 percent chance that a penicillin-allergic individual will be unable to use a cephalosporin without developing an allergic reaction. Whichever antibiotic is chosen, it must be taken for ten to fourteen days, and possibly for a longer period if the sinus problem is more chronic.

Antihistamines and Decongestants. Decongestants include oral medications such as pseudoephedrine (Sudafed) or phenylpropanolamine (Propagest). Often decongestants are used in combination with an antihistamine, although some doctors prefer to avoid antihistamines because they tend to dry secretions and inhibit drainage. Topical nasal decongestants such as Afrin, Neo-Synephrine, and Otrivin have their place in sinus management, as long as they are used under your doctor's instructions in order to avoid rebound nasal congestion.

Steroid Nasal Sprays. Steroid nasal sprays such as flunisolide (Nasalide) or beclomethasone (Beconase or Vancenase) can be tried to reduce inflammation and to bring about decongestion of the nose. Often an over-the-counter nasal spray is used in combination with a steroid nasal spray to shrink the mucus membranes first and allow the steroid spray better access to the nose. This also prevents the potential of rebound nasal congestion, which is often associated with the nasal decongestant sprays when used alone. Typically, the steroid nasal sprays are used for chronic sinus problems, or when an antibiotic has been used with an oral decongestant with little success.

Practical Suggestions. Techniques such as inhaling steam through the nose several times during the day will help to liquefy nasal secretions and promote better drainage. In addition, drinking lots of clear fluids (not milk) will also be of benefit. Airplane travel, swimming, and diving should be avoided. For sinus pain, acetaminophen (Tylenol) is usually sufficient; if not, you should notify your doctor, as a stronger pain medication can be tried. Aspirin-containing products and the cross-reacting medications are best avoided by asthma patients, especially those patients who have nasal polyps (page 34).

Sinus Surgery. Consultation with an otolaryngologist (ear, nose, and throat doctor) is important to check for any anatomical reasons for your sinus problem. In addition, consideration should be given to the possibility of a surgical remedy for your sinus problem if a trial of medical therapy does not resolve it. Surgery can provide larger openings in the sinuses for better drainage (an antral window procedure), as well as clean the sinuses by removing any infected material from the sinus walls (a Caldwell-Luc procedure). If surgery is recommended, your asthma doctor must be involved so that he can reorganize your medications in preparation for surgery, especially if you use steroids on a routine basis.

Sinusitis Should Not Be Ignored. Untreated sinusitis can result in complications such as infection of the bones surrounding the sinus (osteomyelitis), and infection which results in swelling of the eye sockets. Sinus infections need to be treated promptly to prevent the development of chronic sinusitis.

Improvement in Asthma Symptoms. Treatment aimed at resolving the sinus infection and decongesting the nose usually is sufficient to improve asthma symptoms, but more intensive courses of medical therapy or surgery may be necessary. In many cases, improvement in sinus symptoms allows patients who are steroid-dependent to be able to reduce their steroid dose significantly or discontinue using steroids altogether. Any asthma patient who has difficult-to-manage asthma should have a sinus X-ray to check for the possibility of sinusitis, regardless of medical history.

SUMMARY: THE IMPACT OF THE UPPER AIRWAY (NOSE AND SINUSES) ON ASTHMA

1. Congestion in the nose and in the sinuses can be one of the underlying factors that causes asthma symptoms to flare. An examination of your upper airway (including your nose and throat) is an important part of your asthma evaluation.

2. Allergies are just one of the causes of chronic nasal congestion. Other causes include abuse of over-the-counter nasal sprays, hormonal factors such as pregnancy and hypothyroidism, deviation of the nasal septum, nasal polyps, and vasomotor rhinitis.

3. Allergic rhinitis is the medical term used to describe the nasal congestion, runny nose, and sneezing that result from exposure to an allergen such as ragweed or grass pollen. Allergic rhinitis can occur on a seasonal basis (seasonal allergic rhinitis or hay fever) due to exposure to pollen, or on a year-round basis (perennial allergic rhinitis) usually due to exposure to dust, mold, feathers, or animal dander.

4. Both allergic rhinitis and asthma due to allergies are triggered by action of the mast cells and specific IgE antibodies (page 19). The mechanism in both cases is the same, but allergic rhinitis affects the nose while asthma due to allergies affects the airways. With allergic rhinitis, it is important to identify the allergens to which you are sensitive. This is accomplished with the use of allergy skin tests which are compared to your allergic history to make the proper diagnosis.

5. Treatment of allergic rhinitis involves avoidance of the offending allergen if possible, medications to relieve symp-

toms, and a program of allergy shots if indicated. Medication choices include antihistamines (which tend to dry the secretions), decongestants (which make the nose less stuffy), steroid nasal sprays (which reduce inflammation within the nose and make the nose less stuffy), and nasal cromolyn sodium (which serves as a preventative).

6. Allergy immunotherapy (shots) can be very successful in reducing your allergy symptoms so that you need less medication. The greatest success with allergy shots is with patients who are allergic to the seasonal pollens, especially ragweed. Allergy shots take time to work and are most effective in high dosages. Allergy shots must be administered with care and you must be observed for twenty minutes afterward, as reactions can occur which vary from local swelling to a severe reaction called anaphylaxis.

7. Nasal polyps are fluid-filled sacs that arise from the mucus membranes of the nose. All asthma patients who have nasal polyps must be aware that their asthma symptoms may flare with use of aspirin. Aspirin-containing products and the cross-reacting medications should be avoided (page 34).

8. Medical management of nasal polyps relies on the use of topical nasal steroids, antihistamines, decongestants and, when necessary, oral steroids used sparingly. Surgical treatment is often necessary if the polyps cause severe nasal obstruction, although the polyps typically recur within six months of surgery.

9. Sinusitis is inflammation and infection within the sinus cavity. Do not neglect nasal congestion when sinus symptoms flare, since nasal congestion can interfere with the normal drainage of the sinuses.

10. Sinus symptoms can be a subtle factor contributing to asthma symptoms. This most likely occurs when nerves leading from the sinuses and the back of the throat to the airways are stimulated, causing the airways to constrict.

11. Symptoms typical of sinusitis include pressure over the affected sinus area resulting in headache, along with a change in nasal mucus color from clear to yellow or green. The headache is usually worse when first getting up in the morning and when bending down. Fever may or may not occur. An X-ray of the sinuses may be necessary to show clearly the extent of the sinus problem.

12. Medical management of sinus disease includes the use of antibiotics, decongestants, nasal sprays containing topical decongestants (used sparingly under your doctor's guidance to prevent rebound nasal congestion), and topical nasal sprays containing steroid. Practical suggestions such as inhaling steam and drinking lots of clear fluids can help to liquefy your nasal and sinus secretions and to clear blocked nasal passages. Airplane travel, swimming, and diving should be avoided when you have sinus symptoms, unless approved by your doctor.

13. Sinus surgery to ensure proper drainage (antral window procedure) and to clean the sinuses (Caldwell-Luc procedure) should be considered if medical management proves unrewarding.

14. Sinusitis should not be ignored, as complications can occur such as infection of the bones of the sinus and swelling of the eye socket.

15. The possibility of subtle sinus disease should be considered in all patients who have difficult-to-manage asthma, even if they have no symptoms that suggest sinus problems. Improvement in sinus symptoms often helps to eliminate or reduce the asthma patient's need for steroid medications.

◇ **18** ◇

Some Conditions That Can Masquerade as Asthma

Other medical problems can mimic asthma, sometimes making the correct diagnosis much more difficult. Frequent follow-up visits with your asthma doctor in the early stages of treatment will help confirm that asthma is in fact the correct diagnosis. A brief overview of several of the potential problems that can be confused with asthma are presented below.

Distinguishing Asthma from Chronic Bronchitis or Emphysema. The distinction between asthma and chronic bronchitis or emphysema can at times be somewhat confusing, as each condition can cause airway obstruction (measured with a spirometer) that improves somewhat with the use of bronchodilating medications. The patient's medical history is often the best clue in distinguishing asthma from these conditions.

The hallmark of asthma is highly sensitive "irritable" airways, with airway obstruction triggered not just by allergens but by a variety of stimuli, such as cigarette smoke, viral infections, exercise, and cold air. Usually there is marked improvement in airway function after use of a bronchodilating medication. Asthma patients usually describe days when they are free of asthma symptoms as well as days when asthma is out of control. This variability in the extent of airway ob-

struction is typical of an asthma history. Review of the factors
that trigger asthma symptoms (Chapter 2) will provide clues
to suggest whether a patient has asthma, chronic bronchitis,
or emphysema. For example, if a patient has an allergic medical history and positive allergy skin test results and experiences airway obstruction only in the spring and fall, this favors
the diagnosis of asthma on a seasonal allergic basis. This
description of some of the diagnostic clues for asthma is presented to distinguish asthma from chronic bronchitis and emphysema, which are described below.

Chronic Bronchitis. Chronic bronchitis is best defined as
coughing on a daily basis that produces excessive amounts of
mucus from the chest in the early morning hours. Usually the
patient has a history of cigarette smoking. In the later stages
of the disease, shortness of breath occurs in association with
the coughing. Frequently, the mucus becomes infected and
the patient must be treated with antibiotics. Although there
is usually an improvement in symptoms with the use of bronchodilators, some of the blockage within the airways is often
irreversible with chronic bronchitis.

The diagnosis of chronic bronchitis is usually made by
careful evaluation of the patient's medical history (especially
concerning cigarette smoking) in light of the patient's physical examination. The presence of airway obstruction is determined by spirometry. The chest X-ray of a person with
chronic bronchitis can be normal in appearance, although
some linear streaks can at times be seen. Therapy is directed
toward opening the airways as best as possible and treating
any associated infections. Without question, cigarette smoking must be discontinued so that the damage does not progress any further.

Emphysema. Emphysema is a destructive process involving the walls of the air sacs (see Figure 1–1). The damage to
the air sacs caused by emphysema is permanent (unlike
asthma, in which the effect on the airways can be totally reversible). Patients with emphysema usually experience little
coughing. The major symptom is shortness of breath, especially with exercise, that can become progressively worse over

time. A history of cigarette smoking is typical. However, occupational or environmental exposures at work or at home (page 232), or a congenital predilection for emphysema (called alpha$_1$-antitrypsin deficiency) may help to explain emphysema in the nonsmoker. Patients with emphysema often breathe abnormally fast in an effort to maintain the oxygen level in their blood, which often gives their skin a pinkish appearance.

The diagnosis of emphysema is suggested when the patient has a history of shortness of breath that has become progressively worse, along with a long-standing history of cigarette smoking. With emphysema, the patient's chest X-ray may indicate that the lungs are overinflated. Spirometry usually reveals airway obstruction which shows little improvement after use of a bronchodilator, even if a short course of steroids is also taken. Another indication of emphysema is that the oxygen level in the patient's arterial blood decreases with exercise. A breathing test called a diffusion capacity (DLCO) helps to confirm the diagnosis of emphysema.

The treatment of emphysema involves the use of bronchodilators to open the airways as best as possible, antibiotics for any associated infections, a physical therapy program with emphasis on breathing exercises and techniques, and supplemental oxygen if required. Needless to say, cigarette smoking must be discontinued.

Cardiac Asthma. Cardiac asthma is the term used to describe asthmalike symptoms due to heart failure. This condition tends to occur in elderly patients. Often the patients have no history of asthma and these symptoms are a completely new problem. Patients with cardiac asthma do wheeze, but the wheezing occurs as a result of a build-up of fluid in the lungs due to the failure of the heart to pump blood effectively. In addition to a chest examination, there are several clues that doctors look for if they suspect that a patient is in heart failure, such as enlargement of the heart and liver, distention of the veins in the neck, and swelling of the ankles. In some patients, heart failure is diagnosed when a chest X-ray reveals that the heart is enlarged and there is fluid in the lungs. At times, however, there are no clues and the diagnosis is more difficult to make.

The correct diagnosis is important because the therapeutic approach for cardiac asthma is different from routine asthma treatment. Diuretics are often used to reduce the fluid that has built up in the lungs. If this treatment is successful, the problem with wheezing is often resolved.

Pulmonary Embolism. On rare occasion, patients who are thought to have asthma are later discovered to have blood clots that completely or partially obstruct the flow of blood to the lungs. As a result of chemicals released from the cells within the clot, constriction of the airways occurs. In this situation, the patient may have many of the same symptoms as someone who has asthma. Usually there is an obvious medical problem, such as thrombophlebitis (blood clots in the legs), which provides a clue that the problem is not asthma. However, it is possible for a patient to be misdiagnosed as having asthma, when in fact the patient has multiple small pulmonary emboli which are undetected. The correct diagnosis can be difficult.

The diagnosis is ultimately made with either a lung scan (using radio-contrast material to detect areas in the lung that have altered blood flow) or pulmonary angiography (where a catheter is placed into the pulmonary artery so that injected radio-contrast media can be used to view the pulmonary arteries). Pulmonary emboli are treated with anticoagulants to thin the blood rather than asthma medications.

Allergic Bronchopulmonary Aspergillosis. Allergic bronchopulmonary aspergillosis causes wheezing and other symptoms typical of asthma. It occurs as a result of the proliferation within the airways of spores from a mold called Aspergillus fumigatus, and can be a complication of asthma. Patients with this condition often report coughing up brownish mucus plugs. In addition to wheezing, patients complain of achiness, fatigue, and low-grade temperatures. Although microscopic examination of the patient's sputum (mucus from the chest) might reveal the fungus, this does not necessarily confirm the diagnosis as the fungus might be present in patients who do not have this condition.

The diagnosis is confirmed with clues from a series of tests including chest X-ray, spirometry, blood studies, and skin tests. Although allergic bronchopulmonary aspergillosis is more common in Great Britain than in the United States, it does occur in the United States and is often considered as a possible explanation for persistent asthma symptoms.

The primary treatment of allergic bronchopulmonary aspergillosis is steroid medication, with the length of treatment varying from patient to patient. Other asthma medications are often used as well, including theophylline, Adrenalin-like bronchodilators, and cromolyn sodium. Treatment is essential to prevent permanent damage to the lungs, which may occur over time if the condition is left untreated. Allergy shots are not recommended for treatment of allergic bronchopulmonary aspergillosis.

Parasitic Diseases. Any of a variety of parasites can invade the body and cause an infection. Some types of parasites migrate into the lungs and can cause asthma symptoms. Often the clue to diagnosis in this case is a history of foreign travel, or of a previous parasitic infection that may have been incompletely treated. In rare cases the offending parasite can be traced to a household pet.

The diagnosis of a parasitic infection is made by checking a sample of the patient's stool for evidence of the parasite or its eggs. Blood tests can also be helpful in making the diagnosis. The patient's chest X-ray may be abnormal. The treatment is directed to eliminating and killing the specific parasite, usually with oral medications.

Upper Airway Obstruction. Any blockage in the upper airway can cause a wheezing sound that radiates to the chest. However, on careful examination, you or your doctor may notice that the wheezing is actually coming from the neck area rather than from your chest. This observation can be quite important, for it is possible for wheezing such as this to be caused by a polyp on the vocal cord, an enlarged thyroid, or a foreign body such as trapped food. If there is a question in this regard, an otolaryngologist should be consulted for a careful examination of your upper airways.

The diagnosis of an upper airway problem can be made by inserting a thin tube with a light through the nose and into the throat, so that the otolaryngologist can carefully examine your airway from your nose to your vocal cords. This is called a fiber-optic examination of the upper airway. In addition, an X-ray of the neck is sometimes performed to determine if any signs of obstruction are visible. Treatment of an upper airway obstruction depends upon the particular finding, but a surgical remedy for the obstruction may be possible.

The Basic Tests Needed to Confirm the Diagnosis of Asthma.
Along with the medical history and physical exam, spirometry helps to confirm the diagnosis of asthma if it reveals blockage in the airway that can then be reversed with the use of a brochodilating inhaler. As mentioned previously, it is possible for an asthma patient to have a normal spirometry result on any given day. If this is the case, it may be necessary to repeat the spirometry when the person is having asthma symptoms.

The patient's chest X-ray should be checked. The doctor will decide when the chest X-ray should be obtained, taking into account the patient's age, medical history, and the date of any previous X-rays. If asthma is a new problem and the patient has not had a chest X-ray within the last six months, a chest X-ray should be obtained, especially if the patient is an adult who smokes cigarettes. In rare cases, the chest X-ray reveals lung cancer in a patient who has symptoms similar to asthma.

Blood studies often ordered by the doctor to be certain that there is no other medical problem include a complete blood count (to check for an elevation in white blood cells called eosinophils, which tend to be high in allergic individuals), a sedimentation rate (to rule out an inflammatory process such as vasculitis, which at times can mimic asthma), and an IgE level (to check for allergy, if your allergy history is in question). Beyond these basic tests, the patient's medical history will determine if additional studies are necessary, such as allergy skin tests and examination of the upper airways.

If There Is a Question in Your Mind About the Diagnosis, Get a Second Opinion. If there is a question in your mind whether asthma is truly the cause of your problem, mention this to your doctor. A discussion of your concerns and of the reasoning behind the diagnosis may be all that is necessary. If there is still a question, ask your doctor for the name of a board-certified allergist or pulmonary specialist in your community for a second opinion. As an alternative, if you have a local medical school, you can make an appointment for an evaluation by one of the doctors in the allergy or pulmonary sections. The Asthma and Allergy Foundation of America, which may have a local chapter in your area, can also suggest the names of qualified specialists. The National Jewish Center for Immunology and Respiratory Medicine in Denver, Colorado, offers a toll-free hot line to answer questions about asthma: 1-800-222-LUNG.

◇ 19 ◇

Adverse Effects of Oral Steroids

Steroids prescribed for routine use should be added to an asthma treatment plan only when nonsteroid medications have proved unrewarding by themselves. Steroids can be a lifesaving medication when asthma is out of control. All asthma patients must understand that the risk of steroid side effects typically is linked with long-term use of oral steroids, not with short-term use for acute asthma flares. An erroneous concern for steroidal side effects often prevents the use of steroids for controlling acute, difficult-to-manage asthma, with the result that asthma symptoms can progress to a potentially life-threatening point. I cannot emphasize enough that if oral steroids are needed for short-term use to control a difficult asthma flare, the potential benefit of taking the steroids clearly outweighs the small risk of side effects. On the other hand, all asthma patients should be aware of the potential consequences of using oral steroids over a period of months to years. Every effort should be made to reduce the steroid dose to the smallest amount necessary to control the asthma symptoms. Steroids should be taken in as ideal a manner as possible (page 110). If there is no alternative to the prolonged use of oral steroids, the potential side effects should be clearly understood.

Steroids used in asthma management are man-made replications of one of the steroids produced by the adrenal gland. Although the body's steroids help to reduce inflammation, the body does not release a sufficient amount of steroids to relieve asthma symptoms when they occur. Steroids prescribed for asthma treatment are taken in amounts sufficient to reduce inflammation of the airway and to allow the nonsteroid asthma medications to work more effectively. A wide variety of side effects can occur from the use of supplemental steroids. This is easily understood when one considers that the body's adrenal steroids have impact on a myriad of body functions. Table 3–15 highlights the more common potential steroid side effects (page 109).

Weight Gain and Change in Fat Distribution. One of the early effects of oral steroid use is that the face becomes rounder. This is referred to as a moon face. In addition, steroids stimulate the appetite so that weight gain is likely. When steroids are used for a prolonged period, a shift in the distribution of fat occurs. Fat becomes localized in the back in particular, often to the point that the back takes on a "buffalo hump" appearance, as it is called. In contrast, the legs appear thin and wasted. If steroids can be reduced or discontinued, these changes are partially reversible. Fullness of the face caused by steroids is clearly reduced as steroids are tapered.

Osteoporosis. Although many of the steroid side effects are reversible, osteoporosis is irreversible and one of the most serious consequences of long-term steroid therapy. Our bones are continuously being reconditioned throughout life, with bone breakdown and new bone formation occurring constantly. In the elderly, and particularly in the postmenopausal female, there appears to be excessive bone breakdown with less new bone formation. When steroids are taken over a period of months to years, this same pattern favoring breakdown of bone mass occurs. The result is osteoporosis, or weakening of the bones. The exact mechanism explaining how and why osteoporosis occurs in the elderly as well as in those who take steroids is not fully understood.

GREATER CHANCE OF FRACTURES. The concern with osteoporosis is that it increases the likelihood of bone fractures. The weakened bones are unable to resist stress as well as normal bones can. Fractures can occur without significant impact or trauma. Sudden body movements alone have been known to cause fractures when osteoporosis is present. The most frequent complaint with osteoporosis is back pain, which sometimes is the result of fractures of the vertebrae, the skeletal support system of the body. Often the back pain associated with vertebral collapse radiates to the chest or stomach. Collapse of the vertebrae can contribute to curvature of the spine and also to a loss in height. Fractures related to osteoporosis can also occur in the long bones such as the hips, arms, or legs. Ankle and wrist fractures have also been linked to osteoporosis. Therefore, if you have been taking steroids for a prolonged period and you experience any unusual pain in your bones or your back, you should notify your doctor.

X-RAY, THE ONLY DIAGNOSTIC TOOL. Doctors make the diagnosis of osteoporosis by examining your X-rays. Osteoporosis often is first detected when the doctor looks at the spine on a routine chest X-ray and notices that the bones appear less dense than normal. By the time osteoporosis is visible on an X-ray, the condition is in all probability fairly extensive. There is no other test that can detect osteoporosis earlier, although osteoporosis centers utilizing the new technique, photon absorption densitometry, offer promise. However, even if reduced bone mass is not seen on an X-ray, osteoporosis might still be taking place.

POTENTIALLY REVERSIBLE IN CHILDREN, IRREVERSIBLE IN ADULTS. Osteoporosis in children is potentially reversible, as children's bones are frequently and rapidly undergoing new bone formation. The potential does exist that their bones can be strengthened as steroids are reduced or discontinued. In adults, it is unlikely that osteoporosis can be reversed. This has been attempted at several medical centers worldwide; however, there is no clear evidence to date that any treatment for osteoporosis is successful other than reducing steroids when possible.

EFFECTS OF OSTEOPOROSIS SEEN MORE OFTEN IN ELDERLY ADULTS. As mentioned, the elderly are likely to have osteoporosis even when not taking steroids. When oral steroids are taken over a period of time, there is no doubt that the likelihood of developing osteoporosis is increased. Younger patients who take steroids long-term tend to have less problem in this regard, probably because they have greater bone mass which protects them for a longer period from the changes of osteoporosis. Even when osteoporosis does take place in a younger patient, the process often remains undetected until more advanced stages because the dense bone mass of a young person usually obscures the X-ray findings.

TREATMENT FOR OSTEOPOROSIS. There are to date no routine measures to prevent osteoporosis from developing in patients on long-term oral steroids. If vertebral fractures and vertebral collapse have been a problem, back braces and corsets can be used. Heavy lifting and exercises with sudden movements should be avoided. You should also consult an orthopedic surgeon or a rheumatologist for additional suggestions.

CALCIUM, FLUORIDE, VITAMIN D, AND ESTROGENS. Several medication regimens have been tried in the hope of increasing new bone formation once problems have appeared with osteoporosis. Although it would seem that additional calcium should strengthen bones and trigger new bone formation, this has not been the case. Other regimens have been tried, combining various products with the hope of leading to new bone formation. These products include estrogens, calcium, vitamin D, and fluoride.

Estrogens taken by postmenopausal women tend to decrease bone breakdown. They do not, however, increase new bone formation. Therefore, estrogens are most helpful in reducing osteoporosis before it begins in postmenopausal women. Estrogens alone will not increase bone mass in patients on steroids. Calcium has been given in high doses to patients with osteoporosis and has been shown to be of only temporary benefit. At best, calcium supplementation can help partially to arrest osteoporosis, although it will not by itself help to strengthen or create new bone mass. Vitamin D is often given with calcium to improve calcium absorption from the gastrointestinal tract. The addition of fluoride to a regimen of calcium, Vitamin D, and estrogen has also proved beneficial in some patients with osteoporosis. Fluoride becomes incorporated into bones, helping to stabilize them, and may also stimulate new bone formation. This is under study.

Without question, these supplements should be used only with your doctor's advice, as side effects can occur. For example, calcium supplementation can often irritate the stomach and lead to abdominal pain. Vitamin D supplementation in excess can lead to kidney stones and kidney failure in some individuals. Oftentimes, an endocrinologist is consulted for the most updated suggestions in the management of this difficult disorder. To date, there is no truly successful treatment regimen for osteoporosis.

Growth Retardation in Children. When steroids are needed by a child over a prolonged period of months or years, close observation of the child's pattern of growth is important. The child's doctor will keep a record of the child's height and correlate it with growth charts to determine whether the expected rate of growth has occurred. Above all, the doctor should frequently reassess whether steroids are still essential and be certain that steroids are taken in as ideal a manner as possible. In this way the potentially irreversible side effects of long-term steroid use can be avoided or minimized.

Increased Blood Sugar. Steroids tend to elevate the blood sugar. Thus, the use of steroids by the diabetic patient must be closely monitored. An individual with the tendency toward diabetes may develop clear-cut blood sugar elevations when on steroids; in such a case, the steroids have brought out a latent tendency to diabetes that was already present. When steroids are discontinued, the blood sugar levels return to normal ranges in most cases. In individuals with no diabetic tendency, the rise in blood sugar caused by steroids is handled by the body and is not a problem.

Changes in the Skin. Acne is a common side effect of steroid use which often resolves itself without special management once steroids are discontinued. However, a dermatologist should be consulted if this condition persists. If erythromycin is prescribed by the dermatologist, notify your asthma doctor as an adjustment in your theophylline dose may be necessary.

Patients who take steroids on a long-term basis typically develop thinning of the skin. In addition, the small blood vessels located just under the skin become quite fragile. As a result, the skin is easily bruised and takes far longer than usual to heal when injured. The skin of a person using oral steroids for a prolonged period is often analogized to tissue paper because of its thinness and ease in tearing.

Because steroids can act as weak male hormones, the development of finely textured hair, especially about the face and arms, is not unusual during long-term steroid therapy. A consultation with a dermatologist concerning cosmetic approaches can be helpful in such a case.

By far the most displeasing of the skin changes, especially in younger patients, is the development of purplish stretch marks, especially on the abdomen. This occurs as a result of weakening of the supporting tissues under the skin so that the underlying blood vessels are most apparent.

Frequently, all of these changes in the skin improve as the steroid dose is reduced.

Muscle Wasting. The routine use of oral steroids can bring about a gradual reduction of muscle mass. As the first indication one might initially notice muscle weakness. It is possible for muscle weakness to progress to the point where getting out of a chair is difficult and walking is impossible. This tends to occur more severely with the long-acting steroid products such as dexamethasone and triamcinolone, as opposed to the short-acting products. This condition typically reverses itself when steroids are discontinued.

Cataracts and Glaucoma. Cataracts are common side effects of both oral steroids and topical steroids applied to the eye. When changes occur in the lens of the eye such that the lens becomes cloudy, this is called a cataract. Cataracts typically develop in the elderly, but children can develop cataracts with long-term oral steroid use. Increased eye pressure resulting in glaucoma is possible in both children and adults. A careful eye examination by an ophthalmologist should be performed routinely if oral steroids are needed over a long period.

Decreased Resistance to Infection. One of the reasons steroids are used in asthma is to reduce inflammation of the airways. As mentioned previously, steroids prevent the cells involved in the inflammatory process from effectively proceeding to the areas of inflammation. However, the cells that contribute to inflammation are the same cells that afford us protection from infections. Asthma doctors speculate that this is why asthma patients on steroids are more susceptible to infections of all kinds, including viral, bacterial, and fungal infections. If you are taking steroids and you notice any signs of infection, such as a fever or a change in mucus color to yellow or green, you should notify your doctor as soon as possible. Antibiotics are of benefit with bacterial infections only; viral infections do not respond to the available antibiotics. Antibiotics are often prescribed without any sign of infection when asthma symptoms have been long-standing, in order to help clear infected mucus plugs.

The Importance of a Tuberculin Test. A tuberculin skin test called a PPD should, if possible, be performed on all asthma patients before oral steroids are begun. This test tells your doctor if you have been exposed to the organism that causes tuberculosis. A positive test result does not mean that you have tuberculosis, simply that you have been exposed. The diagnosis is made by examining your chest X-ray and culturing your sputum (mucus coughed up from your chest) to determine whether the germ that causes tuberculosis is present. If your tuberculin test is positive and you require routine oral steroids, consideration can be given to administering a medication called isoniazid (INH) to prevent tuberculosis from occurring. If you require routine steroids, and you have a history of tuberculosis or if your tuberculin test has been positive, you should notify your asthma doctor.

Risk of Ulcers. Whether long-term steroid use can cause stomach ulcers is a matter of debate among doctors. There is no doubt, however, that steroids can lead to irritation of the lining of the esophagus and stomach. Steroids should therefore be taken with food. If you have a history of stomach ulcers, the risk of irritation to the stomach from steroids is increased. Patients with supposed steroid-induced ulcers tend to experience abdominal pain in the upper abdomen just below the rib cage. The pain is often described as gnawing. It is also possible that bleeding from the ulcer or perforation of the stomach wall could occur. Therefore, if you have used steroids for a prolonged period and you have stomach pains or notice a change in your stool color (to black, indicating the presence of blood), you should notify your doctor immediately. It is also possible for pancreatitis (inflammation of the pancreas) to cause ulcerlike symptoms.

Salt Retention While Using Steroids. Swelling, especially of the ankles, can occur while taking steroids. This is called edema. As previously mentioned, the presence of adrenal steroids favors salt retention. When salt is retained by the body, water accumulates with it, causing edema. This is an easily managed problem, often remedied by the use of an occasional diuretic if steroids cannot be discontinued. This same mechanism of salt and fluid retention helps to explain the rise in blood pressure that often occurs with steroid use. Here as well, diuretic therapy is often helpful as a simple first step.

When salt is retained, potassium is excreted by the kidneys. Thus, supplemental potassium may sometimes be necessary for patients on high-dose steroid therapy. A low potassium level in the blood may be the reason for the fatigue or listlessness experienced by some patients while taking steroids. If you have any of these symptoms, you should bring them to your doctor's attention.

Endocrine Changes. Steroids may cause irregular menstrual cycles. Once steroids are discontinued, the menstrual cycle often returns to normal. If your menstrual cycle becomes irregular while taking steroids, mention this change to your doctor so that he can rule out any other possibility as the cause. In adolescents, steroid therapy can result in delayed sexual maturation.

Hypothalamic-Pituitary-Adrenal Axis Suppression.
As discussed previously, the use of steroids leads to suppression of the HPA axis (page 106). The extent of the suppression and the length of time it takes for the HPA axis to recover are often dependent on the amount and duration of steroid therapy. Because of suppression of the HPA axis, the adrenal gland is unable to secrete additional steroids needed in times of stress. Therefore, if you require surgery or have an infection, notify your doctor immediately as a large dose of steroids (a steroid boost) is a must. Surgery without additional steroids could be life threatening for a patient who has routinely used steroids within the past year.

Changes in Mood.
When patients begin using steroids, they often feel a sense of euphoria. With long-term use, mood swings from euphoria to depression can occur. Often these changes in mood correspond to steroid dosage changes. Reassurance often is sufficient to manage this problem but some patients will need the support of psychiatric counseling, especially if there is little likelihood that a steroid dosage adjustment is possible.

Fear of Steroid Side Effects Should Not Discourage Steroid Use When Truly Necessary.
Although steroids can be associated with many potential side effects, their use is essential for some patients with severe asthma. In such cases, fear of steroid side effects should not discourage their use, since asthma can be a life-threatening illness if left untreated. If your doctor has determined that routine, long-term use of oral steroids is necessary to manage your asthma, steroids should be taken in as ideal a manner as possible to reduce the risk of side effects.

PART SIX

◇◇◇◇◇

Conclusion

◇ 20 ◇

Final Summary

Asthma is a chronic illness which cannot be cured but can be well managed. Successful management requires that you be well informed. With the background about asthma provided in this book, along with an explicit, written asthma treatment plan prepared with your doctor (including instructions as to when to contact your doctor), most asthma patients can manage their asthma themselves on a day-to-day basis. By being prepared in advance, a flare of asthma symptoms will not take you by surprise, and can be promptly and appropriately treated. I believe that this method of dealing with asthma will reduce the need for frequent emergency visits to the doctor's office or to the hospital.

The concept of self-management requires your participation to be certain that you clearly understand: (a) the factors that trigger your asthma symptoms; (b) the logic for deciding whether you need asthma medications on a daily basis or only when your asthma flares; (c) how to use the prescribed medications properly; and (d) when to notify your doctor if your treatment plan does not seem to be controlling your asthma. Asthma is best treated promptly. It would be a mistake to think that the concept of self-management in any way implies that you should ever struggle on your own with asthma symptoms—for example, overusing an inhaler or taking extra med-

---

Some Myths about Asthma

* Asthma is "all in your head"

* Asthma is always due to allergy

* Asthma leads to emphysema

* Asthma is always cured by moving to another geographical location

* Asthma is never a cause of death

Table 20-1

ication that has not been recommended by your doctor. Self-management is possible only if you are committed to following the specific instructions of your doctor and notifying him if the proposed plan fails to control your asthma promptly.

Table 20–1 presents some of the common myths about asthma that have been clarified in previous chapters. A list of the essential points stressed in this book follows.

1. Asthma is best described as reversible obstructive airway disease. The airway obstruction results from constriction of the muscles surrounding the airways, swelling and inflammation of the lining of the air tubes, and increased mucus production. The blockage in the airways can usually be reversed with proper medications. The airway obstruction can be confirmed with the use of a breathing test called spirometry.

2. Asthma affects the airways, not the air sacs, and is reversible. Asthma does not lead to emphysema, which involves the air sacs and is irreversible.

3. The hallmark of asthma is "twitchy airways," which are ready to constrict at any time in response to any of several different factors.

4. Asthma usually occurs in attacks spaced by symptom-

free intervals, but it may also occur on a continuous basis. Asthma symptoms can vary and are not limited to wheezing but may include only a subtle cough. In order to understand better your own asthma history, refer to Table 1-1, "Developing Your Asthma Case History."

5. Although the tendency to develop asthma does have a genetic basis, the exact cause of asthma is not known. However, there are several major factors that can trigger asthma attacks: infections, allergy, aspirin and aspirin-containing products as well as yellow food dye #5, exercise, emotional upset, irritants, and foods (rarely). Be sure you know which are the key factors that affect your asthma.

6. Not everyone who has asthma is allergic. Allergy is but one of the factors that can trigger asthma symptoms. The pattern and timing of your asthma symptoms can provide clues suggesting that allergy may be causing your asthma. Seasonal asthma symptoms suggest that a seasonal pollen is the culprit; year-round asthma symptoms can be caused by dust, molds, animal dander, and feathers. The question of whether allergens affect your asthma can be clarified by seeing an allergist and having allergy skin testing. Treatment of allergies consists of avoidance of the offending allergen as much as possible, judicious use of medication to relieve the symptoms, and allergy immunotherapy (shots) when appropriate.

7. Viral infections (such as colds) are more likely to cause asthma symptoms than bacterial infections (such as strep throat). Underlying sinus problems can make asthma symptoms more difficult to manage. If asthma symptoms persist beyond a few days, mucus plugging your airways could become infected, thereby delaying the resolution of your asthma symptoms. Notify your doctor promptly if you have any signs of an underlying infection.

8. Exercise can trigger asthma symptoms in many individuals with asthma, but this does not mean that people with

asthma should not or cannot exercise. Exercise-induced asthma can be well managed with the use of pretreatment medications taken before exercise begins. Asthma patients should know that activities that involve brief intervals of exercise (such as baseball, golf, and football), as well as certain other exercises (such as swimming), are less likely to provoke asthma symptoms. See Table 2–2 for a checklist of practical suggestions.

9. Aspirin and products that contain aspirin can trigger asthma attacks in certain individuals. Aspirin can trigger attacks which come on quite suddenly (within minutes), or make asthma attacks more difficult to manage. Aspirin-sensitive patients should also avoid the cross-reacting medications, such as nonsteroidal anti-inflammatory medications and yellow food dye #5 (see Table 2–4). Because aspirin can trigger asthma symptoms in as many as one out of every five asthma patients, regardless of their prior experience with aspirin, many doctors suggest that aspirin is best avoided by all asthma patients, since acetaminophen (Tylenol) is an acceptable alternative.

10. All patients who have nasal polyps should strictly avoid aspirin-containing products and products that cross-react with aspirin. Triad asthma is the combination of nasal polyps, asthma, and aspirin sensitivity.

11. Irritants such as cigarette smoke and cold air can directly trigger asthma symptoms. The asthma symptoms are not caused by an allergy to the irritant but rather by the irritating effect on the patient's airways. Newer inhaled medications, available by prescription, are fast-acting and are the best choice of medication in this situation.

12. Asthma is not a psychosomatic illness. Emotional upset can, however, make asthma symptoms worse. If this is the case, emotional aspects of your asthma should be considered in your asthma management plan.

13. Although foods can trigger asthma symptoms, current

evidence suggests that foods are an infrequent cause of routine asthma symptoms. Children are often placed on milk-free or wheat-free diets to see if there is any improvement in asthma symptoms. Attention has recently focused on the association between food additives (such as sulfites and yellow food dye #5) and asthma symptoms in some asthma patients. As some asthma medications contain sulfites, it is important to review this question with your doctor.

14. The basis for most asthma treatment plans involves the use of medications. Patients are often surprised to learn that there are but four major categories of asthma medications: theophylline products, Adrenalin-like bronchodilators, cromolyn sodium, and steroids. Details are provided in individual chapters on the effect and proper use of each of these medications.

15. The goal of any asthma treatment plan is twofold—to minimize the impact of asthma on one's day-to-day life, through the use of an asthma medication plan and avoidance regimen carefully designed with your doctor, and, when appropriate, a program of allergy shots; and to avoid the need for steroids or to reduce the use of steroids to the minimal amount necessary, administered in the safest way possible.

16. Adrenalin (epinephrine) is usually the first medication used for asthma that is out of control. Adrenalin works by rapidly opening the airways. Adrenalin side effects include accelerated heart rate, shakiness, nausea, and vomiting; these side effects usually are transient. Doctors often give two Adrenalin shots spaced by twenty minutes, as the effect of Adrenalin wears off quickly. A long-acting form of Adrenalin called Sus-phrine is often used once wheezing has subsided, to keep the airways open until other medications take effect. As an alternative to Adrenalin, an inhalation treatment can be given via a nebulizer using Bronkosol or Alupent. This is usually associated with less side effects than Adrenalin.

17. Newer medications similar to Adrenalin offer the advantage of rapid opening of the airways along with the convenience of oral and/or inhaled methods of use. The newer medications provide more direct action on the lungs with less effect on the heart than Adrenalin, as well as a longer duration of action. Products such as albuterol (Proventil or Ventolin), terbutaline (Brethine, Bricanyl, or Brethaire), or metaproterenol (Alupent or Metaprel) are examples of the category of medications referred to in this text as the Adrenalin-like bronchodilators.

18. Asthma inhalers act directly on the airways, with less risk of the side effects often associated with oral asthma medications. Proper inhaler technique is important to derive the greatest possible benefit from inhaled medications. Inhalers must never be overused. If you find that you are using your inhaler more frequently than recommended, call your doctor so as not to delay any necessary additional therapy or emergency treatment.

19. Theophylline relaxes the muscles surrounding the air tubes, helping to relieve asthma symptoms. There is no standard dose of theophylline correct for everyone. Therefore, the proper dose of theophylline must be determined on an individual basis. This is done through the use of a blood test called a theophylline level.

20. Potential side effects of theophylline include nausea, headache, diarrhea, and jitteriness. If you have any of these symptoms, notify your doctor as your dosage of theophylline may need to be decreased. Remember that the addition of certain medications, such as the antibiotic erythromycin, may necessitate an adjustment in your theophylline dose.

21. The choice between a long-acting and a short-acting theophylline product depends on your asthma history. Long-acting theophylline offers the convenience of an eight-to-twelve hour interval between doses, so that you can have an uninterrupted night of sleep. Theophylline prod-

ucts lasting twenty-four hours are also available and are appropriate for some people. The short-acting products act more rapidly, and are more appropriate for individuals who need rapid relief and have infrequent asthma symptoms.

22. Cromolyn is an often-overlooked asthma medication that deserves serious consideration in any asthma program. It is an inhaled product and an effective pretreatment for exercise-induced asthma, cold air-induced asthma, and asthma triggered by a foreseeable exposure to an allergen such as animal dander. Since it is a preventative medication, cromolyn will not control asthma symptoms when they flare. It is essentially free of side effects in most individuals.

23. Oral steroids are the last medication to be added to an asthma medication program. For routine use, the benefit achieved in managing asthma with the use of steroids must be weighed against the potential risks associated with its long-term use. Side effects with the long-term use of steroids can include osteoporosis, high blood pressure, diabetes, cataracts, and growth retardation in children. A more complete list of potential steroid side effects is presented in Table 3-15.

24. The risk with oral steroids, even in high doses, is not with occasional short-term use but rather with their long-term use. Short courses of oral steroids, even in high doses, can be used with little risk of side effects. Oral steroids should be started early during severe asthma episodes that are unresponsive to the nonsteroid medications, as steroids take four to six hours to work. For difficult-to-manage asthma, steroids can be a lifesaving medication.

25. If oral steroids are needed for a prolonged period to keep asthma under control, using them in an ideal manner can reduce the risk of developing side effects. The most preferable way to use oral steroids on a long-term basis in-

cludes: (a) use of steroids early in the morning, preferably every other day, as opposed to use in both the morning and the evening; (b) use of shorter acting steroid preparations such as prednisone, prednisolone, or methylprednisolone, as opposed to longer acting agents such as injected or oral dexamethasone or triamcinolone; and (c) use of the least amount of steroids necessary to control asthma symptoms, taken as infrequently as possible.

26. Inhaled steroids offer the advantage of acting directly at the site of the problem (the airways) with less absorption of steroid into the body. Often the oral steroid dose can be reduced or discontinued with the addition of inhaled steroids. Inhaled steroids are preventative agents—they do not offer immediate relief of asthma symptoms. Inhaled steroids have only a small risk of steroid side effects. The major side effect of inhaled steroids is thrush.

27. For patients who take steroids on a routine basis, or have taken steroids intermittently over the past year, the steroid dose must be increased during times of stress (such as an infection or surgery).

28. Decisions regarding steroid dosages should be made by the doctor caring for your asthma.

29. There are other medications that can be used for special circumstances in asthma management, such as atropine and troleandomycin. TaO is reserved for patients who require high dosages of oral steroids on a routine basis. TaO should be used under the direction of a doctor familiar with its use and potential side effects.

30. An asthma treatment plan with a written medication program, either prepared by your doctor or prepared by you in accordance with your doctor's instructions, is essential for successful self-management of your asthma. If you write your own plan from what your doctor has told you, bring it with you to your next visit so that your doctor

can review it. Be certain to discuss at what point he wants you to notify him if your asthma symptoms flare.

31. Ask your doctor if he recommends a peak-flow meter to measure your lung function at home, a spacing device to assist in better inhalation technique, or a nebulizer unit to deliver an inhalation treatment at home (using Alupent or Bronkosol).

32. Be sure that all of your doctors and your dentist know that you have asthma.

33. Avoid the group of medications called the beta blockers (such as Inderal), as they have been associated with triggering asthma symptoms. Beta blockers are sometimes used in eye drops for glaucoma.

34. Sedatives or sleeping pills must never be used when you are having asthma symptoms. This is a firm rule.

35. Suggestions for reducing your exposure to allergens and irritants to which you are sensitive may seem burdensome, but such measures clearly have been shown to help reduce asthma symptoms. Particular attention should be paid to making your bedroom a haven from allergens such as dust and molds, and irritants such as perfumes, hair sprays, and cigarette smoke.

36. Allergy shots, which are small doses of the allergen(s) to which you are sensitive, help to reduce your sensitivity to the injected allergens over time. The goal with an allergy shot program is to reduce your need for medications and to reduce your symptoms. Accurate diagnostic testing is essential in order for the allergy shot program to be most effective. The highest success rate with allergy shots is with the seasonal pollens.

37. The estimate of the number of American children with asthma is between 5 and 10 percent. Asthma is the most common cause of school absenteeism of the chronic ill-

nesses affecting children. Approximately 50 percent of all children with asthma "outgrow" their asthma by age fifteen; no doubt the increase in the size of the airways as the child matures is a contributing factor.

38. Treatment of asthma in children is similar to treatment of adults with asthma. Key differences include: (a) special attention to the theophylline dose, using blood theophylline levels as a guide, as young children tend to rapidly metabolize theophylline; (b) use of preventative medications such as cromolyn sodium (Intal), which is essentially free of side effects; (c) use of special devices for inhaled medications, including inhalation chambers, spacing devices, nebulizers, and whistle attachments; (d) a plan to manage attacks that in children can begin quite suddenly. Awareness of asthma self-management is as important for the child as for the parent.

39. Asthma that is well managed and free of complications has little effect on pregnancy, as there are no clear-cut consequences from asthma during pregnancy for either the mother or the fetus. If asthma medications are necessary during pregnancy, they must be reviewed with your asthma doctor as well as with your obstetrician. Several of the theophylline products, bronchodilating inhalers, and even steroids (if there is no alternative) can be used during pregnancy when necessary, with little risk of side effect to the fetus. Asthma medications that should be avoided during pregnancy are summarized in Table 9–1.

40. Exposure to offending agents in the work place can sometimes trigger asthma symptoms. Asthma flares can occur immediately or on a delayed basis, several hours after exposure. Occupations associated with a potential asthma risk are listed in Table 10–1. There is a risk of serious, irreversible airway obstruction associated with long-term occupational asthma. This emphasizes the importance of prompt diagnosis along with periodic breath-

ing tests and preexposure medications, with consideration given to a change of work environment, if appropriate.

41. When an asthma patient requires surgery, coordination is necessary among the surgeon, the anesthesiologist, and the doctor caring for your asthma. Depending on the type of procedure and the choice of anesthesia, adjustments in your asthma medications may be required. A steroid boost may be necessary if you have taken steroids during the last twelve months.

42. If your asthma is made worse by emotional upset, various psychologically oriented approaches may be helpful, such as biofeedback, hypnosis, family counseling, educational seminars, and psychotherapy. It is important to think of yourself not as an asthmatic but as a person who has asthma.

43. A clear-cut explanation of why asthma symptoms tend to flare at night and in the early morning hours is not yet available. Long-acting theophylline is the preferable medication for routine nighttime asthma symptoms. Possible underlying causes that should be considered include subtle sinus symptoms, postnasal drip, and gastroesophageal reflux.

44. Not everyone who wheezes has asthma. For example, elderly patients who wheeze may have underlying heart problems termed "cardiac asthma." In addition to a history and physical examination, basic tests needed to confirm the diagnosis of asthma include spirometry and a chest X-ray. Blood studies such as a complete blood count, a sedimentation rate, and allergy skin tests may also be helpful if indicated by your medical history.

45. Status asthmaticus is a severe, potentially life-threatening asthma episode that initially fails to respond to routine treatment, including Adrenalin (and/or an inhaled bronchodilator) and intravenous theophylline. Steroids are essential during status asthmaticus. The goal once

asthma symptoms are under control is to avoid a recurrence of status asthmaticus.

46. You are an essential part of the management team. You must be able to identify asthma symptoms early so that they can be promptly treated. Do not ignore asthma symptoms that fail to respond to recommended medications. Prescribed medications must be taken as directed and on time. Be sure that you do not break any of the rules recommended by your doctor including: (a) Do not use sleeping pills or sedatives with asthma symptoms. (b) Do not overuse your inhaler. (c) Never alter your theophylline or steroid doses on your own. (d) If you are sensitive to them, be diligent in avoiding aspirin-containing products, nonsteroidal anti-inflammatories, tartrazine (yellow food dye #5), and sulfites. A written medication program will help you coordinate these instructions.

47. When asthma symptoms are difficult to manage, asthma doctors often check for any underlying problems such as unsuspected sinusitis or gastroesophageal reflux. In addition, doctors often review the points outlined in Table 20–2, as attention to detail is the key to managing difficult asthma.

48. The impact of the nose and upper airway on the lower airways must be considered in all asthma patients. Polyps on the vocal cords can sometimes masquerade as asthma. An examination by an otolaryngologist can be helpful to determine whether there is an upper airway problem.

49. Allergic rhinitis (hay fever), nasal polyps, and sinusitis can all have impact on asthma. Improvement of upper airway problems often makes asthma management easier.

The importance of a good working relationship with your doctor cannot be overemphasized. A medication plan that

Points Sometimes Overlooked in Asthma Care

1. Determining the ideal dose of theophylline for each person, since theophylline requirements can vary up to sevenfold from person to person.

2. Fine-tuning of the theophylline dose by obtaining appropriately timed (peak or trough) theophylline levels.

3. Demonstrating proper inhaler technique and following up to be sure that the patient is using the inhaler correctly.

4. Being sure that the patient understands the potential risks of inhaler overuse.

5. Timing the patient's medications to be most effective when symptoms are most likely to occur.

6. Treating upper airway problems (such as sinus infections or hay fever) which may contribute to asthma symptoms.

7. Using a pretreatment regimen to allow the asthma patient to be able to exercise rather than discouraging him from exercising.

8. Considering the use of a preventative medication (such as cromolyn sodium or inhaled steroids) to be used routinely to avert daily asthma symptoms, rather than relying on routine oral steroids.

9. Taking steroids as a single morning dose (if possible) as opposed to taking a split daily dose (in the morning and evening).

Table 20–2

allows you a measure of self-management is important to reduce the fear and confusion that can be associated with an asthma flare. Self-management is effective as long as you clearly understand that your doctor must know if your medications are not working or if your asthma is out of control.

Modifications in your medication program may be necessary, so give your doctor the chance to know if the suggestions initially presented have not been fully effective.

If your asthma is still out of control after modifications of your program and you frequently wind up in the emergency room, you might wish to contact the university medical center closest to you. The National Jewish Center for Immunology and Respiratory Medicine in Denver, Colorado (one of the major asthma and allergy centers in the United States), maintains a hot line staffed by nurses to answer questions concerning asthma. In addition, they often can provide the name of a specialist in asthma in your area of the country. The toll-free number is (800) 222-LUNG. Other sources of information about asthma can be found in Appendix B.

Above all else, do not be afraid to tell your doctor that you are concerned about your asthma and would like a second opinion. Doctors want the best for their patients and rarely object to their patients seeking a second opinion.

This book can serve as a starting point for a better understanding of your asthma. My patients often share with me their insights and suggestions about their asthma. This has helped me to better help them and other asthma patients. As no two asthma patients are alike, I invite you to share your thoughts and comments with me so that with subsequent editions, this book will grow and continue to improve. Also, updates on the latest research, medications, and products, as well as practical suggestions, are presented in *The Asthma and Allergy Update*, a monthly newsletter of which I am one of the editors. To obtain further information or to share your suggestions with me, you can write to: *The Asthma and Allergy Update*, P. O. Box 34735, Bethesda, Maryland, 20817.

◇ Appendix A ◇

Pollen Calendar
of the United States

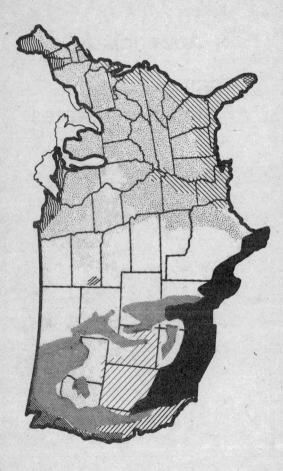

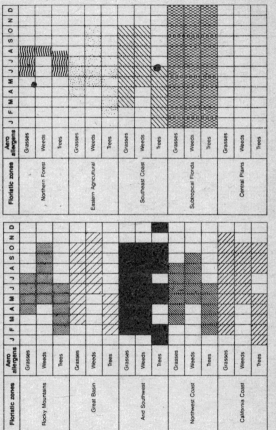

Adapted from The Journal of Respiratory Diseases 6(8):60-61. 1985. Copyright © 1985. Cliggott Publishing Co

◇ Appendix B ◇

Sources for Further Information

The following is a listing of national organizations that provide informational assistance to individuals with asthma and/or allergies.

Asthma and Allergy Foundation of America
National Headquarters
1717 Massachusetts Avenue, N.W.
Suite 305
Washington, DC 20036

American Lung Association
1740 Broadway
New York, NY 10019

National Heart, Lung and Blood Institute
National Institutes of Health
Building 31
9000 Rockville Pike
Bethesda, MD 20892

National Institute of Allergy
and Infectious Diseases
National Institutes of Health
Building 31
9000 Rockville Pike
Bethesda, MD 20892

National Jewish Center for Immunology
and Respiratory Medicine
(formerly National Jewish Hospital/
National Asthma Center)
1400 Jackson Street
Denver, CO 80206

American Academy of Allergy and Immunology
611 East Wells Street
Milwaukee, WI 53202

American College of Allergists
800 East Northwest Highway
Mount Prospect, IL 60056

American Association for Clinical Immunology
and Allergy
P.O. Box 912
Omaha, NE 68101

American Society of Internal Medicine
2550 M Street, N.W.
Washington, DC 20037

American Academy of Pediatrics
P.O. Box 1034
Evanston, IL 60204

Mothers of Asthmatics
5316 Summit Drive
Fairfax, VA 22030

◇ Index ◇

◇ About the Author ◇

Allan M. Weinstein, M.D. is a board-certified allergist who practices in Washington, D.C. ASTHMA is the result of the author's years of clinical experience with children and adults at the National Asthma Center in Denver, consulting with the National Institutes of Health, and his private practice. Dr. Weinstein is an Assistant Clinical Professor of Medicine at Georgetown University. He is a member of the American Academy of Allergy and Immunology, and a medical advisor to the Asthma & Allergy Foundation of America.

Dr. Weinstein lives in Maryland with his wife and family.

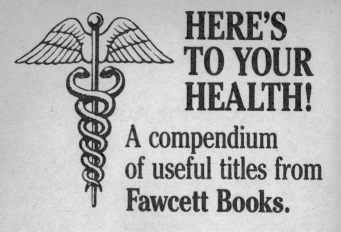

HERE'S TO YOUR HEALTH!

A compendium of useful titles from Fawcett Books.